The

LITTLE BOOK

of

THIN

The

LITTLE BOOK

of

THIN

FOODTRAINERS™

*Plan-It-to-Lose-It Solutions
for Every Diet Dilemma*

LAUREN SLAYTON, MS, RD

A PERIGEE BOOK

A PERIGEE BOOK
Published by the Penguin Group
Penguin Group (USA) LLC
375 Hudson Street, New York, New York 10014

USA • Canada • UK • Ireland • Australia • New Zealand • India • South Africa • China

penguin.com

A Penguin Random House Company

Library of Congress Cataloging-in-Publication Data

Slayton, Lauren.
The little book of thin : Foodtrainers plan-it-to-lose-it solutions for every
diet dilemma / Lauren Slayton, MS, RD.
pages   cm
Includes index.
ISBN 978-0-399-16600-6 (pbk.)
1. Reducing diets.   2. Nutrition.   3. Compulsive eating—Prevention.   I. Title.
RM222.2.S575   2013
613.2'5—dc23   2013032621

First edition: January 2014

PRINTED IN THE UNITED STATES OF AMERICA
10   9   8   7   6   5   4   3   2

To Marc, Myles, and Weston for embracing sprouted bread, smoothies, and me.

CONTENTS

THINTRODUCTION   ix

1. Ten Steps to Svelte   1

2. Breakup Time   12

3. LBT What-to-Eat Cheat Sheet   20

4. Skinny Starts Sunday   32

5. The Witching Hour   49

6. Treat Training   66

7. Family Style   76

8. Restaurant "Reservations"   84

9. Living Social   97

10. Are Your Workouts Working for You?   112

11. Trimming Your Travel   121

12. Pre-Beach Procedures, aka the Drastic Chapter   133

13. Holy Holiday Hazards   143

14. Thintastically Ever After   158

LBT RECIPES   165

LBT LINGO   193

LBT NO-ROLL-ODEX   197

ACKNOWLEDGMENTS   201

INDEX   203

THINTRODUCTION

A goal without a plan is just a wish.

—ANTOINE DE SAINT-EXUPÉRY

Congratulations; I hear you're ready to graduate from dieting as you know it. Whether it's the silly balls behind the ears, couscous only, baby food, the HCG diet, or cleansing, we're all susceptible to diet hype. I have popped whole cloves of garlic and tried sword-fighting workouts because I heard they worked or I hoped they would. Inevitably, like you, I've asked myself, "What was I thinking?"

A few things can be gleaned from the fact that the average dieter makes four attempts at weight loss a year. The optimist in me admires the tenacity. I take a couple of stabs at finding a missing glove and soon acknowledge it just might never be found. That said, four attempts also indicate that multiple diets or plans are failing. And that's per year. What about dieters who try to lose weight year after year? Does that really mean eight or twelve or more plans have failed them over time?

In initial sessions with new Foodtrainers clients, I ask about these previous forays into the diet world, as well as what did, and didn't, work for them. Sometimes I hear, "Weight Watchers is good for portion control" or "I liked

South Beach; I do better with fewer carbs." My favorite answer to this question came from a tough-cookie real estate broker who looked me in the eye and said, "Lauren, obviously nothing has worked or I wouldn't be here." It was up to me to solve this client's diet dilemmas, and I did. Now I'm here to guide you through your final diet.

After years of nutrition counseling, it's easy for me to see where most food plans fall short. Whether it's low carb or high fiber, portion control or vegan, almost all diets focus on food choices. Can you imagine if a therapist said to you, "Here is a list of ways you should think. If you follow this list you'll be happy." That sounds ludicrous (I hope). Diets that are based solely on food lists are exactly the same thing. But no matter how many diets you've tried, research shows perpetual dieters are not doomed. You are just as likely to shed pounds as diet virgins. *The Little Book of Thin* will help you figure out what really works—for you, for the long term.

The key to successful weight loss is to know the diet strategies for various circumstances. What happens to your eating when you travel? Or when you bring an after-school snack for your kids but nothing for yourself? How do you make sure you don't arrive home after work and raid the fridge with your coat still on, keys in hand? If nutrition knowledge equaled weight loss, we would all be thin. We know what to eat until life gets in the way.

Winging It Doesn't Work for Weight Loss

When you wing it, you end up with the bagel at the breakfast meeting or the candy bowl in the afternoon. Believe it or not, more diets are lost because of a hectic schedule than an extra treat.

At Foodtrainers, I "train" clients to develop a skill set for tackling food challenges. I am a nutrition trouble-shooter who has seen every possible situation that can sabotage even the most dedicated dieter. These challenges are not isolated to birthdays and holidays; for most people, frenzied is the norm. In this book, I share the strategies and tips to avoid the most common diet booby traps. You will learn what I consider to be the most valuable long-term weight loss lessons that will enable you to plan and prepare, and even to veer occasionally from your course—and still succeed.

Personal chefs and meal plans with prepared food work because you don't have to make food decisions. However, when you make food decisions in advance, you become the personal chef for a whole lot less money. The money saved? You can use it for new skinny clothes; perhaps a little black dress (LBD) after completing *The Little Book of Thin* (LBT).

The missing component in diet success is planning and anticipating food obstacles. Starting with the basics—the Ten Steps to Svelte and a short list of no-no's—and moving on to Smart Snacks and my Pre-Beach Procedures, you'll find dozens of hints and tips to see you through the most common diet challenges. Most importantly, you'll develop new thin habits that you can live with. Foodtraining is not about sentencing you to life without your favorite foods, or curtailing your social schedule. Life's too short to cry over a caramel or a cocktail. Weight loss takes work but you don't need to feel deprived, choke down things you dislike, or live without the occasional indulgence. You certainly don't have to be overweight or unhappy. You just have to Plan-It-to-Lose-It!

One

Ten Steps to Svelte

*Good habits, once established, are just
as hard to break as are bad habits.*
—ROBERT PULLER

Over the past decade, I've developed individualized food plans for thousands of clients, but as different as these plans might be, I always start my counseling sessions with the essentials, or what I call the Ten Steps to Svelte. Whether you are single or a senior, already health conscious or nutritionally challenged, the following are absolute do-not-pass-go crucial behaviors that *everyone* should establish. They provide the guideposts you can rely on when life gets crazy—or crazier than normal.

Forget about the constant, often conflicting, nutrition information twitting about in your brain. It's time to simplify things. Organizing your Ten Steps to Svelte prepares you for weight loss success. My team at Foodtrainers recently conducted a six-week program at an investment firm. Before we started with one-on-one sessions, we gave all the participants homework: increase their hydration, exercise effectively (only 100 minutes per week to start), and sleep seven hours a night. We thought they might think we were wasting their time with such rudimentary requests. But when we weighed them after the first week, thirty-one out of thirty-three newbie Foodtrainees had lost weight.

When you get your essentials in order, you feel confident and in control and you can tackle other areas of your eating. Sure, there's a part of every one of us that craves quick and extreme results. We'll get to "drastic" (Chapter 12, "Pre-Beach Procedures"), but we have to be strategic about it. First, you need to follow the Ten Steps to Svelte and refine the day-to-day behaviors that are holding you back.

1. Eat a Protein Breakfast Within Two Hours of Waking Up

Not everyone is hungry the second they wake up. It's fine to wait a bit before eating—but not too long. If you wait too long to eat, your blood sugar will drop and you'll be starving later in the day. You can't catch up if this happens, because even once you eat you'll feel unsatisfied. Timing is definitely one of the most underestimated ingredients for weight loss. At the start of each day, adhere to a firm two-hour rule: if you're up at 7 a.m., have breakfast by 9.

Protein helps control your cravings and appetite. At the

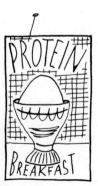

risk of being a nutrition nerd, let me introduce you to *ghrelin* because if you're trying to lose weight, the hormone ghrelin is the enemy. This "hunger" hormone makes you crave calorie-dense foods (to remember ghrelin's function, I think, ghrelin makes you "growl"). A study in the *American Journal of Clinical Nutrition* confirmed that eating some form of protein at the start of the day will keep nasty ghrelin at bay. Good-bye, ghrelin—jerk!

2. Take Supplements of Omega-3 and Vitamin D

I don't think most healthy people should take handfuls of vitamins a day. If you're eating correctly, you don't need to. I do believe almost everyone should take two supplements: omega-3s and vitamin D. You probably have heard that omega-3s are heart healthy or anti-inflammatory, but most importantly for dieters, omega-3s increase lipolysis (translation: They help you lose more fat or "inches"). Take at least 1,000 milligrams of omega-3s per day.

If ghrelin is the dietary devil telling you to "eat more," leptin is the appetite angel hormone. Leptin says, *You've had enough, you can stop eating*; love that leptin. Vitamin D and leptin are related. More vitamin D means more leptin. Bottom line: If you have low vitamin D levels, you won't lose weight as quickly. And there's a bonus: Vitamin D also helps regulate mood and overall well-being. Quicker weight loss and better mood: Who can say no to that? Just be sure to take enough vitamin D (1,000– 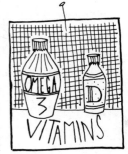 2,000 IU daily) to have the appetite angel, leptin, on your side. There are many "fish" in the omega-3 and vitamin D "sea," but I like the Nordic Naturals brand Ultimate Omega and Carlson Vitamin D3 drops (2,000 IU).

You can find a complete list of all the brands or "names" I name in the LBT No-Roll-odex.

Put your vitamins near your toothbrush to remind you to take them.

3. Drink the Right Things, Skip the Others

During the day, water and tea are all you need!

Drinking water doesn't require great effort, but it sends your body the message you're doing something right, and this can have a carryover effect. Research has shown that drinking 16 ounces of water before each meal or snack is the most effective way to promote weight loss. In one study, participants who drank water in this manner lost 5 additional pounds compared to those who drank the same amount of water but not immediately before a meal. If you're one of many water haters, I recommend Hint Water and Herbal Water, which are flavored but unsweetened. But cucumber slices and sprigs of fresh mint are my favorite DIY hydration helpers.

Green, white, and oolong teas are mild metabolism boosters. Drinking these is the equivalent of burning 50 to 75 extra calories a day. For most of us, that is reason enough to imbibe, but if you need additional incentive, you may have heard that research suggests that green tea is also beneficial in protecting against heart disease and certain cancers. Try 8 to 12 ounces of good-quality tea a day. Freshly brewed is best, but I'm a big fan of Eboost's Pink Lemonade Effervescent Powder, which includes green tea along with other vitamins, minerals, and supernutrients.

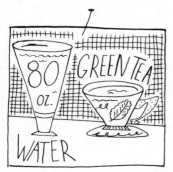

Your Water Bottle May Be Making You Fat

More and more studies are concluding that there are endocrine-disrupting chemicals in such wide-ranging items as personal care products, canned goods, and many forms of plastic. You may have heard of BPA (bisphenol A—I know, science again); this is just one example of a hormone disrupter we come in contact with. These chemicals, known as *obesogens*, can affect the size of your fat cells and fat storage. The FDA has banned BPAs in baby bottles and sippy cups, but adults have been left to play "sippy roulette." To minimize exposure to these chemicals that affect your weight—and your risk of cancer too—use glass water bottles.

4. Eat Four Fish Meals a Week

I mentioned the benefit of omega-3s earlier, and while omega-3 supplements are important, you also want to get some of your omega-3s from food. Fish eating will make a difference in your weight loss results.

While salmon gets the attention, all fish have some omega-3s. In the course of a week, choose fish for four or more meals. The best eco-friendly seafood picks for weight loss, other than wild salmon, are char, black cod, mussels, oysters, and those little fishies, sardines and anchovies. Some trusted sources

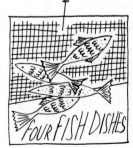

for fish are Tonnino jarred tuna, Vital Choice Salmon, and Cole's sardines.

5. Enjoy One Fruit Daily—But No More

Fruit is the best "sweet" there is. Fruit provides fiber, vitamins, and fluid. Fruit also "doles out" sugar, and you know what happens to excess sugar? Yes, it's welcomed warmly by your fat cells. *Dieters beware: It is possible to overfruit.* For weight loss, stick to one serving per day. A serving is one cup of cut fruit or a medium piece of fruit. Think baseball, not softball. If you purchase packaged cut fruit, there's usually 2 cups (a pint)—twice the recommended portion. Be sure to save half or share.

The top five Foodtrainers fruits based on calories, fiber, and glycemic load are Asian pears, strawberries, raspberries, papaya, and grapefruit.

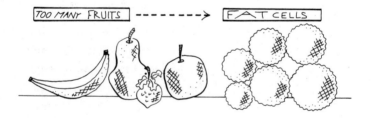

6. Limit Grains, Carbs, and Starchy Vegetables to Once a Day

While I was at a lecture given by Dr. David Ludwig, the obesity expert and professor at Harvard's School of Public Health, he said, "We have no biological requirement for grains." I refrained from shouting "Bravo" from the audience. While we can debate the best or better grains and carbs, the fact is we don't need them. Plus, when you eat fewer grain foods, you automatically eat more vegetables. You may love your bread or pasta, but chances are you need to spend less time together. What has gluten done for you lately? So if you have your oatmeal (in Chapter 3, "LBT What-to-Eat Cheat Sheet," we'll dis-

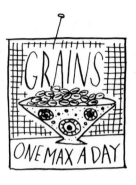

cuss which carbs are LBT legal) in the morning, skip the quinoa at lunch. And if you know you're having a sushi dinner, avoid the carbs earlier in the day. Plan. Plan. Plan-It-to-Lose-It.

7. Let's Do Dunch

Make lunch larger than dinner. Do you eat like a bird all day long if you're going out to dinner? Many people are guilty of "banking" their calories, or saving them up in anticipation of a large evening meal. This sounds semirea-sonable until you find yourself diving into the bread basket and then ordering dessert "to share" with the table. Sud-denly, you've more than made up for the daytime sacrifice.

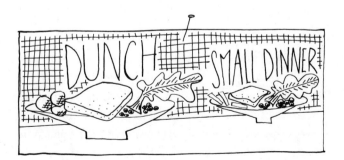

Twice a week of hitting the bread basket and having "bites" of dessert (usually around a quarter of the whole dessert) sadly aggregates to more than 8 pounds a year.

You've heard of breakfast for dinner. My vote is dinner for lunch; I call it "dunch." When you think about it, your midday meal has to energize you for the rest of the day. Dinner just sends you to bed. Which meal do you think should be larger? An entrée at lunch of poached salmon or grilled chicken and a side of green vegetables works well. Despite what you've heard, the important part of breakfast is just making sure you eat *something within two hours of getting up (with protein); it doesn't have to be a large something.* Lunch is the most important meal and can make or break your entire food day. Show lunch some respect.

8. Close the Kitchen After Dinner

Try for twelve food-free hours between dinner and breakfast (see, once again timing is important for weight loss). There's plenty of interesting research that indicates that a "fasting" period of even twelve hours can turn on something call the "skinny" gene (also known as SIRT1), which prevents fat storage inside the body. After the evening meal, dessert just doesn't work, but herbal tea does. And a little

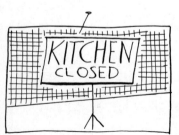

chamomile will also help with another step to svelte, getting a good night's sleep.

Now, if you're going to start the dessert lobby with the maxim, "Everything in moderation," I'll ask how that's been working for you. Who wants to fit into their clothes moderately? Or feel moderately well? You don't; you want to feel thin, so Plan-It thin.

9. Sleep Seven Hours a Night

You're busy. Maybe you wake up as early as 4:30 or 5:00 a.m. to work out, attend to emails, or start a long commute. While this is admirable, it only works if you are also early to bed. Burn the candle at both ends and you may not be so fond of your "end." Those hunger hormones and appetite angels need sleep to recalibrate. Close the kitchen and impose an electronic curfew two 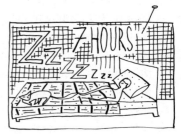 hours before bed—banish the cell phone, tablet, TV, computer, and any other device that may be keeping you mentally stimulated—and heavier than you'd like to be.

10. Get 180 Minutes of Cardio a Week

I don't believe one day makes or breaks anything. There are days you will not exercise or not have time to do 45 minutes or an hour's worth. You can reach the ideal goal of 180 minutes a week of cardio any way you want. This amount of time per week will produce results but doesn't require you to quit your job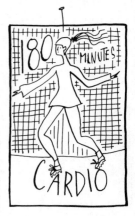

in order to exercise. We'll get to exercise particulars later, but note that exercise is the last of my ten tips for a reason. Exercise on its own will not make you thinner, but exercise and *The Little Book of Thin* will.

The Ten Steps to Svelte—I know you are not doing all of them. (I *know* these things.) Whether it's consuming four fish meals or fitting in your 180 exercise minutes, this is where thin begins. Richard Branson, the CEO of Virgin (who knows a thing or two about success), is a fan of lists and advises, "Mark off every completed task—you'll find making each tick very satisfying." Continually refer to this svelte checklist. Whenever you're not feeling your best, return to this list. Chances are you're neglecting one of the essentials and something's out of whack. Reclaim control, get back on track, and move on.

TEN STEPS TO SVELTE

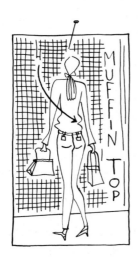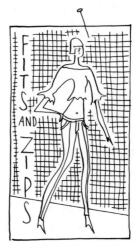

No		Yes
❏	**1.** Eat a protein breakfast within **2** hours of waking up.	❏
❏	**2.** Take supplements of omega-**3**s and vitamin **D**.	❏
❏	**3.** Drink **80** ounces water/seltzer and **2** cups green tea daily.	❏
❏	**4.** Eat at least **4** fish meals a week.	❏
❏	**5.** Enjoy **1** fruit daily—but no more.	❏
❏	**6.** Limit grains, carbs, or starchy vegetables to **once** a day.	❏
❏	**7.** Make lunch **larger** than dinner.	❏
❏	**8.** After dinner, the kitchen is **closed**.	❏
❏	**9.** Sleep **7** hours a night.	❏
❏	**10. 180** minutes of cardio a week.	❏

Two

Breakup Time

I'll probably feel a whole lot better when you're gone.
—TOM PETTY

You've probably noticed that the Ten Steps to Svelte don't involve forgoing many things. Nobody likes to feel deprived. Personally, I love chocolate and cheese and have been known to concoct an insanely good elderflower martini. And believe me, I'm not nibbling on dry arugula as I write. But just as there are Ten Steps to Svelte (outlined on page 11), sometimes you just have to say *No*. So here's a short list of No's to stick to if you absolutely want to slim down starting now.

Before I get to specifics, however, there are three major No's:

- No Negotiation
- No Excuses
- No Exceptions

I realize No's aren't easy, but I've found that firm rules are easier for most people to follow. The minute you start to negotiate with yourself about food, it's a slippery slope. With the No's, there are no exceptions. Chances are, at least a few of the items on the following No list make regular appearances in your life. Foods are a lot like relationships, and it's time to break up with soda, Caesar dressing, and corn flakes. You'll feel better and look better without them holding you back. And because I know change—even when it's for the best—is scary, I have you covered with rebound options.

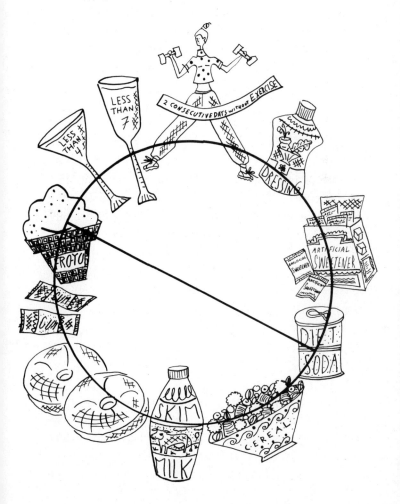

No Soda

Soda (diet included) promotes weight gain, not loss. Sweet begets sweet, and even artificial sweeteners dull taste buds, so they may lead to more intense sweet cravings. There is no way to say which is "better," diet or regular soda; they're both disastrous. Diet soda drinkers have higher levels of abdominal fat, and diet soda, though "sugar-free," has been shown to raise blood sugar levels. Soda = toxic relationship.

On the Rebound: Hint Fizz, Eboost, or Sparkling Herbal Water.

No "Diet" Food

Beware of anything that is labeled sugar-free or fat-free. What stands in for fat and sugar is always problematic. While I know you're not a mouse, one twelve-week study showed that mice that were given artificially sweetened yogurt gained more weight than the critters consuming sugar-sweetened yogurt. Food impostors are not only bad for you; they're bad for your weight. Skip fake anything: artificial sweeteners (the pink, the blue, or the yellow), faux meat (textured vegetable protein), faux butter—anything referred to as a substitute. Diet foods are the smooth talkers, whispering sweet nothings but delivering disappointment.

On the Rebound: Pastured or grass-fed butter (contains conjugated linoleic acid [CLA], which decreases body fat, specifically abdominal fat); NuStevia (a good alternative to artificial sweeteners).

No Skim Dairy

Nonfat dairy may be the ultimate example of dietary infidelity. Many people wasted years on skim milk only to find out it's not what they thought it was.

On the Rebound: Low-fat or 2% yogurt and 2% organic milk.

Fat-Free Can Make You Fatter

In the 1990s we learned that fat-free makes you fatter. My real concern with skim milk was stirred after reading Walter Willett's *Fertility Foods*, in which he explained that the process that removes the fat from milk concentrates androgens (read: male hormones) and other hormones in the remaining portion, adversely affecting fertility. But that's only part of the story . . .

Skim milk doesn't help you lose weight. A study of almost twenty thousand women found that those who increased their skim dairy consumption gained 10 percent over nine years. Yet those who increased whole milk consumption, by even one serving a day, lost 9 percent on average. Fat in milk helps us assimilate vitamin D (recall that low vitamin D = slower weight loss) and keeps us full. It also tempers how the sugars from milk are released into our bloodstream. If you still have lingering fat phobia, just bump yourself up to 1% or 2%. As the great Joan Gussow, food policy pioneer, said, "I trust cows more than chemists." I do too—and I think we've all had enough gray cups of coffee in this lifetime.

No Cold Cereal

For the most part, cold cereal is carby, sweet, and highly processed. Cold cereal is not the breakfast of champions, at least not thin champions. Cold cereal can be likened to a first crush. As innocent as it seems, it rarely continues into adulthood, or if it does, it probably shouldn't. If you are telling yourself you're having cold cereal for the fiber, there are much more wholesome fiber sources.

On the Rebound: Cocomama Quinoa Cereal and Vigilant Eats oat-based cereal cups (which can be eaten cold or hot and bring something to the table other than simple sugars and carbs). Remember, if you have cereal for breakfast, that's your one "good grain" for the day.

No Bagels

Many clients have been scarred by my saying: "Bagels aren't for thin people," but it's important to know that a bagel is equal to five slices of bread. Bagels are akin to the relationship that isn't perfect but it's easy, predictable, and readily available. With food and love, ubiquity isn't usually healthy. In general, when it comes to bread, spending a little time breadless never hurt anyone.

On the Rebound: Orgran Multigrain Crispibread with Quinoa or sprouted bread.

No Frozen Yogurt

Fro-yo is a friend with benefits, a no-strings-attached relationship. It seems great to think you can have dessert and lose weight. Then you realize you're not losing weight. At most frozen yogurt shops the portions, even those called "small," are way too big. Plus, once you have that massive cup, the topping temptation is hard to pass up.

On the Rebound: While I think it's risky to eat after dinner, if you want a sweet, frozen something, it's acceptable to "meet up" midafternoon. Almond Dream makes adorable "bites." I also like Coconut Bliss pops from Luna and Larry's. These pops have good ingredients and reliable, fixed portions, and there's no candy sprinkled on top.

No Bottled Salad Dressing

You've gone to the trouble of getting (or bringing) a salad for lunch and now you're going to coat it in sugar and salt? I'm guessing you wouldn't put two to three teaspoons of sugar on a salad. For some dressings it's not even sugar (or something wholesome like maple syrup) but sucralose or corn syrup. Bottled salad dressing is a commitment-phobic food. Why not let yourself be both healthy and thin? You don't have to sabotage your efforts.

On the Rebound: Make your own dressing. (See Thin-I-Gette Dressing, page 181.)

No Gum

Gum makes you gassy; gum contains multiple artificial sweeteners, preservatives, and food dyes. Plus, gum chewing doesn't look nice. Gum is the promiscuous person's food. Part of losing weight is realizing we don't always have to have something in our mouths.

On the Rebound: Sweet Riot chocolate-covered cacao nibs will take the lunch taste out of your mouth; parsley is a natural breath mint. And keeping a toothbrush in your makeup case is calorie free.

Gum Ingredient Labels: Reading the Fine Print

Sorbitol is sugar alcohol, aka guaranteed gassiness.

Gum base

Glycerol

Mannitol is another sugar alcohol; bystanders beware.

Natural and artificial flavors

Hydrogenated starch hydrolysates (also called polyols) are 20 to 50 percent as sweet as sugar.

Aspartame (less than 2 percent) is a migraine trigger, carcinogen, and potential contributor to preterm labor.

Acesulfame K stimulates insulin secretion, part of the argument that sweet begets sweet. Plus, it hasn't been properly tested.

Soy lecithin (an emulsifier) is separated from soybean oil by the use of chemical solvents; plus, should we place bets about whether this soy has not been genetically modified (GM)?

BHT is used to maintain freshness; it is banned in England. At higher doses it has been shown to cause animals to bleed in the brain. It can damage heart cells and retard weight gain.

Colors such as Blue 1 Lake. Blue 1 Lake has been shown to cause brain tumors in animals.

No More Than Four Alcoholic Drinks a Week for Women/ No More Than Seven for Men

Clients often ask, "If I'm doing most things right, do alcohol calories count?" It turns out they do, and your body will not burn anything else until it gets rid of your cocktails. Think of liquor like flirting. It all counts and if you cross the line, you'll be in trouble.

On the Rebound: Plan-It-to-Lose-It by setting a limit for the number of drinks you will have before you start drinking—and stick with it. (In Chapter 8, "Restaurant 'Reservations,'" we'll get specific about *what* to drink.)

No More Than Two Consecutive Days Without Exercise

Exercise is similar to marriage. If you want to keep a marriage strong, you need to work at it. The more days you go without exercise, the less you'll end up doing.

On the Rebound: Level with yourself; if you skip Monday and Tuesday, Wednesday has to happen.

I will embarrassingly quote Taylor Swift. When it comes to the No list, tell yourself: "We are never, ever getting back together."

Three

LBT What-to-Eat Cheat Sheet

Never eat anything bigger than your head.
—MISS PIGGY

In the previous chapters, we've laid the groundwork for serious weight loss. You're familiar with the Ten Steps to Svelte and you've learned how to survive food breakups. Now we can get to the nitty-gritty of what and how much to eat.

What to Eat

New clients often ask, "Is this okay to eat?" As you know by now, I don't want you to feel just okay. *The Little Book of Thin* is about you feeling your absolute best. In the following sections and the subsequent Cheat Sheet, you'll find what I consider the top choices in each category of food, or the real "skinny."

PROTEIN
Quality is a concern for every food you eat, but nowhere is it more crucial than when selecting meat, poultry, eggs,

and dairy products. The difference between organic and conventional is a matter of what the animals are fed and often whether hormones or antibiotics are administered. Without question, certain hormones, antibiotics, and pesticides may very well affect our weight.

In Chapter 1, I talked about "obesogens" that leach from plastic water bottles. Many other additives and pesticides are also in the obesogen category. If you feel you're doing everything right and not getting results, examine the *quality* of your food and choose organic for poultry, grass-fed for beef, and wild for fish. And of course you can still Plan-It thin if you don't eat meat or poultry. (See the *Little Book of Thin* Cheat Sheet.) You don't have to be anxiety-ridden about selecting food, just be aware.

CARBS

Carbs are so controversial. Let's be blunt: Most people, left to their own devices, would eat too many carbs. Pasta, bread, tortillas, and grainy desserts all make the list of the top ten foods consumed by U.S. adults.

A carb hierarchy exists. Your starchy vegetables, such as sweet potatoes, are whole, unprocessed foods and the best carbs you can eat. When it comes to grains, there's a big difference between wheat and other grains. You will lose weight more efficiently if you eat brown rice or quinoa than if you eat whole wheat (mostly not so "whole") bread. You will not find whole wheat bread on the LBT Cheat Sheet. In fact, the only bread mentioned is sprouted bread (see the "Better Bread" sidebar).

Most of the carbs and snacks on this plan are gluten-free; you don't have to be 100 percent gluten-free, but by virtue of heeding the Cheat Sheet, consider yourself gluten-reduced. You'll also note that legumes—that is, beans, lentils, and chickpeas—count as carbs. Sad, I know, but true.

Better Bread: Why Sprouted Grains Are Different

To make white bread, part of the wheat kernel (the nutritious part) is removed and the remaining portion milled into flour. Sprouted-grain breads use the whole kernel (sort of like a seed), which is allowed to grow slightly but not into a full plant.

Sprouted grains are higher in nutrients than their unsprouted counterparts and easier to digest. Sprouted wheat contains four times the amount of niacin and nearly twice the amount of vitamin B6 and folate. While sprouted wheat is a source of gluten, it is the best source, and some people with gluten issues find they can include sprouted wheat in their diets. One of the key benefits of sprouted-grain products is that they are higher in protein than other breads, and some of the carbohydrates are lost in the process of sprouting.

Since sprouted-grain products are such a departure from their refined and processed counterparts, they are often referred to as "live food." Certain varieties have been deemed acceptable by many raw foodists. Since sprouted grain products are "alive" and perishable, they are best kept in the freezer or the refrigerator, which is why you won't find them in the doughy bread aisle alongside those icky white hot dog buns. My favorite sprouted-grain breads are Food for Life Ezekiel 4:9, Shiloh Farms Organic Sprouted 7 Grain bread, and French Meadow Sprouted 16 Grain and Seed bread.

VEGETABLES

Vegetables are the basis for any healthy food plan and should figure prominently into all your LBT meals. The only ones you need to watch and "count" are your starchy vegetables: sweet potatoes, winter squash, corn, and peas. Other than that, the more, the "thinner," as most vegetables are unlimited. A recent study in *Obesity* showed that fiber was associated with a reduction in belly fat. *Eat green, get lean:* artichokes, asparagus, kale, bok choy, chard, and the healthiest vegetable of all, microgreens, should be on your weekly shopping list.

FRUIT

At Foodtrainers, we created a spreadsheet for clients to compare the amount of fiber, sugar, calories, and glycemic load for all fruits. For example, some fruits may be higher in sugar but low in calories. To simplify things for you, you'll find the fruits that have the best average "score" listed on the LBT Cheat Sheet in this chapter. These are the best all-around weight loss fruits—but don't fall into the trap of overfruiting.

FATS

Fats are an integral component of a healthy diet, and I'm happy to see that fat phobia is almost a thing of the past, a diet relic if you will. Oils such as olive, coconut, and sesame help you absorb fat-soluble nutrients, and when used properly, they improve the weight loss process. "Proper" in this case is a maximum of one tablespoon per meal. We still need to be fat aware, but a small amount of fat will extend the staying power of your meals.

You will probably recognize most of the nuts and seeds on the Cheat Sheet, but there are two with which you may not be familiar: chia seeds and hemp seeds. Both contain omega-3s and fiber. Chia seeds are a natural appetite suppressant, and magnesium-rich hemp seeds are a secret weapon that will help you lose body fat. Sprinkle these seeds in yogurt or over a salad.

Beverages

In Chapter 1, "Ten Steps to Svelte," we discussed the importance of water and green tea. You'll find other calorie-free beverages listed on your LBT Cheat Sheet. The other category, Liquid Snacks, includes coconut water, kombucha, and green juices that are strategic "thin" additions if you stick to a maximum of one from this category per day.

LBT Cheat Sheet

There's a chance your favorite fruit or carb may not appear on the list, but these choices are the most strategic selections I can offer. Stick to this Cheat Sheet and you'll lose weight.

PROTEIN

Whenever possible, choose organic for meat, dairy, and eggs. Aim for four or more fish meals a week.

Beef (grass-fed)	Pork (tenderloin or loin)
Bison	Turkey
Chicken	Yogurt (low-fat or 2%
Eggs (omega-3)	Greek-style)
Kefir	

Hemp protein

Pea protein

Whey (grass-fed)
protein

Arctic char

Black cod

Mussels

Oysters

Salmon (wild; fresh or
smoked)

Sardines

Scallops

Shrimp

Sole

Tuna (fresh or
jarred)

CARBS

One fist-size portion unless otherwise indicated; between three and six portions per week.

Beans

Chickpeas

Corn

Lentils

Oats (not instant)

Quinoa

Rice (black or brown)

Sprouted bread (2 slices)

Sprouted tortilla
(1 tortilla)

Sushi roll (one 6-piece
maki roll)

Sweet potato

Winter squash

VEGETABLES

Eat green. Get lean.

Artichokes

Arugula

Asparagus

Bok choy

Broccoli

Brussels sprouts

Cabbage

Cauliflower

Celery

Chard

Cucumbers

Dandelion greens

Fennel

Garlic

Green beans

Jicama

Kale

Lettuce

Microgreens

Mushrooms

Onions

Peppers

Pickles (lacto-fermented)

Radishes

Spinach

Summer squash
(zucchini)

Tomatoes

FRUIT

One piece or one cup a day. Overfruiting? No way. (Lemon/lime in water doesn't count as your one fruit for the day.)

Apple

Asian pear

Grapefruit

Lemon

Lime

Papaya

Pear

Pineapple

Raspberries

Strawberries

Watermelon

SEEDS, NUTS, AND HEALTHY FATS

Many of these will help you look and feel better, but be mindful of amounts. A tablespoon or a sprinkle is perfect.

Chia seeds

CocoChia (coconut/chia
seed blend)

Almonds

Pecans

Avocados

Hemp seeds

Pumpkin seeds

Sunflower seeds

Pistachios

Walnuts

Butter (pastured)

Coconut oil

Olives

Olive oil (extra virgin)

Sesame oil

SALAD ACCESSORIES

Here's the bling of the food world. A little goes a long way; one "accessory" per salad.

Avocados

Olives

Dried fruit

Seeds

Nuts

CONDIMENTS AND FLAVORINGS

No-calorie and low-calorie choices to add a lot of zing and variety to your meals without the guilt. Go wild.

Cayenne

Lemon juice

Cinnamon

Miso

Crushed red pepper
   flakes

Mustard

NuStevia (sweetener)

Fresh herbs

Turmeric

Ginger

Vinegar

Hot sauce

BEVERAGES

The following count as water, but many have added nutritional bonuses:

Eboost

Teas: green, herbal
   oolong, pu-erh, or
   white

Herbal Water

Hint Water

Matcha (powdered
   green tea)

LIQUID SNACKS

These healthy drinks have a few more calories than other recommended beverages, so stick to one a day maximum:

Coconut water

Green juice

Kombucha (fermented tea)

ALCOHOL

We'll cover cocktails later (see "Be Choosy When You're Boozy," page 92), but in simple terms, have four or fewer drinks per week.

Bourbon

Sake

Scotch

Tequila

Vodka

Wine (red, white, or sparkling)

How Much and How Often to Eat

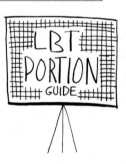

I don't believe in weighing and measuring all your food. It's not the ¼ ounce of chicken or the extra drop of olive oil that will make a difference in the long run. Depending on your dieting history, this statement will sound either emancipating or downright scary. Don't get me wrong, it does matter how much you eat, but you can use common sense to determine the portions that are right for you.

When it comes to portion sizes, perhaps you've heard the old "deck of cards" used as a visual aid; I don't know about you but it has been some time since I played gin rummy. Hopefully my portion references will make more sense.

PROTEIN

Seek out organic grass-fed beef, free-range chicken, and wild fish.

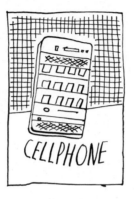

CHEESE

It's hard to resist—but often a nibble of cheese becomes a bite and then . . . I don't think of cheese as an everyday food, but if you want a little snack or to taste-test at a party . . . it's a "lipstick tube" or less.

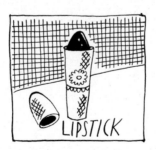

CARBS

I know, I know, everyone's fist is different, but that's the point; it's proportionate to *your* body and probably a smaller portion than you usually take. Choose carbs carefully. (See the LBT Cheat Sheet.)

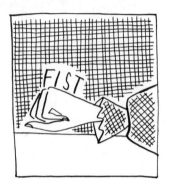

FRUIT

Sure, most fruit is packed with nutrition, but most also has a lot of sugar. Keep in mind that I never recommend fruit juice.

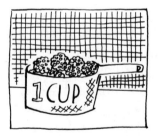

VEGETABLES

At lunch and dinner, aim to have veggies equal to about two cups. Visualize an individual Greek yogurt container for one cup. Vegetables are not just for garnish. Remember, there are exceptions to the "eat more veggies" rule since starchy vegetables are considered carbs.

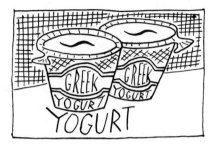

NUTS

These little nuggets have many nutritional virtues but are calorically dense.

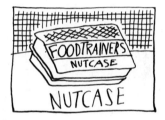

Now that you're familiar with how much to eat, I want to be sure you didn't miss something important on the Cheat Sheet and that's *how often* you should have certain foods. I mentioned that you should have carbs no more than once a day; what you now see is that in a week you will have three to six "fists" of carbs. For drinks you may have four per week. With these budgets in mind, you can look at your calendar for the week and know when you'll be out or when cocktails are most likely. Now that you know the Cheat Sheet, in the next chapter the real planning begins.

Four

Skinny Starts Sunday

An ounce of prevention is worth a pound of cure.
—BEN FRANKLIN

It's 7 p.m. on a weekday and you walk in the door, tired, hungry, and cranky. Looks like it's takeout for dinner (again) . . . We've all been there; it's a pattern we fall into and it's hard to fix midweek. Whether it's the megamuffin at the morning meeting or pad Thai for dinner, you don't want to indulge in something simply because it's there, especially when there's such an easy fix. It's easy to eat correctly when you have the right foods on hand, but you have to set yourself up properly.

My best example of planning for the week ahead comes from an adorable ER doctor client, Dr. O. In our initial session, I heard about her shifts and schedule and felt hives coming on. I introduced her to Skinny Starts Sunday and my 3 P's, which are Plan, Purchase, and Prep. When we met again one week later, Dr. O. proved my concern was unfounded and showed me, once again, that the busiest people are often best at scheduling; they have no choice. Dr. O was able to solve her planning problems by prepping the bulk of the week's meals and bringing her food to eat at the hospital. She didn't have to eat pizza in the break room or vending machine snacks. She also didn't have food rotting in her fridge.

I asked her how she felt once she organized her eating, and she said, "I am in a caregiving profession and give a lot of my physical and emotional energy to strangers. By planning, I am doing something healthy and productive to care for myself. Also, cooking is one area of my life where I have some control. I control the ingredients I buy; I control what I make. No matter what happens, every day I know that by eating my own food, I have done something nice for myself."

If this sounds unimaginable to you, I'm not saying that you have to cook a week's worth of meals at a time. I'm saying that an ounce of prevention is worth a pound of cure (or fat).

A good friend of mine has weight loss items she refers to as "promise foods." Special K is a promise food (it promises it'll make you thin, though it will not). But what if the "promise" didn't come in a box or a capsule but was a behavior that actually lived up to its promise? What I call the 3 P's really work, and when they do, it's gratifying. As Dr. O described, once you get in a cooking groove, it's rewarding to know exactly what's in your food and to nurture yourself.

I know the kitchen can be an intimidating place, but as Mario Batali said, cooking has more to do with finger painting than math; it's okay to color outside of the lines. There's no report card in your kitchen, so don't worry about the outcome. It's impossible to be a healthy, lean person if all your food comes in a box. If you practice these 3 P's, I'm willing to *promise* you that you'll feel better and look better too.

The 3 P's: Plan, Purchase, Prep

STEP 1: PLAN

In your electronic or old-school calendar (nothing wrong with pens and pencils), write "Plan It" on every Sunday for the next month. I like Sundays because many people aren't working and it paves the way for a less manic Monday. If Sundays are out, your planning day can be any day, as long as it's predetermined.

Look at your calendar for the week ahead and make a menu of what you plan to eat for breakfast, lunch, and dinner. You can use our Menu Map (see page 36) as a template to map your weekly menu. Don't panic; I'm going to explain the LBT choices for each meal, but for now I'm just explaining the process. If you normally buy lunch during the workweek, decide what those lunches will be and then write them down. For example, "takeout salad with salmon and avocado." Decide if there's anything you need to skip; for example, on your menu with the salad, also write "no bread." If there are nights you know you will be out for dinner, show that on your Menu Map. Ideally, you want to be cooking more meals than you're eating out.

Just remember that mental decisions do *not* equal an official plan. Don't overcomplicate this; complicated can be a barrier. You can start your menu mapping using the LBT Top Five lists and recipes and of course your Cheat Sheet foods. Keep it simple. A few items in a steady rotation work well. Start with two breakfast choices and two lunch choices per week. Repetition builds rhythm. Sounds boring? Bore yourself thin.

Top Five LBT Breakfasts

Remember to have breakfast within two hours of waking up.

1. 2% Greek or Siggi's low-fat (not nonfat) yogurt with either 2 tablespoons hemp seeds or ½ package CocoChia

   - Greek yogurt has a higher protein content than other yogurt. Siggi's is high in protein but also comes in interesting flavors; it's the only flavored yogurt I recommend. Hemp seeds and CocoChia (a coconut/chia seed probiotic blend) are nutritious mix-ins.

2. Two whole omega-3 eggs (any style) with 1 cup papaya or raspberries

   - Two omega-3 eggs can be paired with any LBT-approved fruit.

3. Two ounces wild smoked salmon *or* 1 to 2 tablespoons almond butter on two Orgran gluten-free crackers

   - This is an easy breakfast option. I recommend Orgran's quinoa crackers.

4. LBT Starter Smoothie (page 177)

   - Make sure you have a strong blender and these key ingredients: protein powder, fresh or frozen fruit, greens, and liquid.

5. Green Eggs Muffin-Tin Frittatas (page 169)

   - These mini frittatas are a great make-ahead egg option using leftover vegetables.

Foodtrainers Menu Map

	SUNDAY	MONDAY	TUESDAY
BREAKFAST			
LUNCH			
SNACK			
DINNER			
VICTORY LIST			

Shopping List

BREAKFAST ITEMS	LUNCH ITEMS	SNACKS ITEMS	DINNER ITEMS
_____	_____	_____	_____
_____	_____	_____	_____
_____	_____	_____	_____
_____	_____	_____	_____
_____	_____	_____	_____
_____	_____	_____	_____

LBT Guide
R: Restaurant (check menu ahead)
T/O: Takeout

WEDNESDAY	THURSDAY	FRIDAY	SATURDAY

LBT Truths

- ❑ Skinny starts Sunday.
- ❑ If it's not on the list, can't buy it.
- ❑ Plan for a green, a grain, and a main.

Top Five LBT Lunches (or "Dunches")

Every lunch should include a minimum of 2 cups of a Cheat Sheet vegetable or greens.

1. Essential Poached Salmon (page 186) with steamed asparagus

   • Poached wild salmon is easy to prepare and delicious served cold.

2. Baby spinach with Tonnino tuna or shrimp

   • I love tuna that comes packed in a jar. It is sold packed in olive oil or water; either is fine. Jarred tuna is more expensive than canned, but you'll get two servings per jar and no obesogens. The salad in this lunch should include only one "accessory," such as half an avocado, walnuts, or olives. Dress with Thin-I-Gette Dressing (see page 181) or 1 tablespoon olive oil and lemon juice or vinegar.

3. "Greek" Curried Chicken Salad (page 173) over mesclun greens

   • The combination of Greek yogurt, anti-inflammatory spices, and greens make this lunch a triple treat nutrition-wise.

4. Pesto Turkey Burgers (page 182) or veggie burgers with roasted cauliflower

   • The turkey burgers should be prepared with organic ground turkey. I recommend only two prepared veggie burger brands: Sunshine or Hilary's.

5. Miso Broccoli and Quinoa Salad (page 167) with sliced cucumbers and celery on the side

- There is no way you feel deprived eating this flavorful salad. Make sure you stick to a one-"fist" portion—and count it as your carb for the day.

Top Five LBT Dinners

All dinners should have a protein, copious vegetables, and an optional Cheat Sheet–approved carb. Dinner should be smaller than lunch. Serve it on a small, salad-size plate to help portion control. And, of course, feel free to use the lunch suggestions for dinner. Whenever possible choose organic meats, grass-fed beef, and wild fish.

1. No-Fuss Fish (page 188) with steamed broccoli

   - This is an easy dish to help reach your four fish meals for the week.

2. Beef and Spinach "Green Balls" (page 185) and steamed green beans

   - These are breadcrumb-free meatballs made with grass-fed beef. Make extra and freeze them.

3. Starter Chicken Cutlets (page 171) and Starter Kale (page 168)

   - There is no reason to order in a grilled chicken salad. DIY and you can choose organic chicken and use extra cutlets for soup or salads during the week.

4. Weekday Tenderloin (page 183) and Kale Slaw (page 170)

   - Can't leave out the other white meat; pork tenderloin is super lean and a nice departure from chicken overload.

5. Loaded Sweet Potato

- Don't get too excited; this is not the loaded potato you may have pictured. It's as delicious as the traditional version, which is loaded with cheese, sour cream, bacon bits, and sundry other things. But it's so much better for you. Simply bake a small sweet potato at 450°F for 45 to 60 minutes, or until tender, cut in half lengthwise, and top with Starter Kale (see page 168), ½ sliced avocado, chopped scallions, and crushed red pepper flakes. Voilà!

STEP 2: PURCHASE

Grocery shopping is something you know how to do, but that doesn't mean you're doing it effectively (most of us don't). When you're shopping systematically, you'll arrive home with bona fide meal components. On the other hand, when you end up with a random assortment of foods with various degrees of healthfulness, you're likely "fat" shopping versus food shopping. Earlier I mentioned that you probably know what foods you should be eating. Let's make sure your cart or basket reflects that.

Success starts before you get to the store. Map your weekly menu and make a shopping list *beforehand* so that you can shop strategically. Ideally, decide on your menu at home so you can see what you already have and what you need to buy. (Even if you find yourself headed to the store menuless, stop and take five minutes to make a menu that can be your guide for shopping. It's not ideal, but it's better than shopping blind.)

Strategic shopping guidelines include the following:

- If it's not on the list, you cannot buy it. Impulse buys typically make up over 50 percent of the grocery bill. Planning can save you both money and calories.

- No "store d'oeuvres," which the Urban Dictionary defines as "snacks and food samples to tempt the patrons into buying something they weren't planning on." The only thing you can munch on while shopping is veggies. Maybe you should hit the produce section first.
- "No impulse buys" applies to other family members; nice try. Do not justify chips by thinking they're for your husband. When they are in your house, suddenly they're for you.
- If it's available to you, online grocery shopping is a great option. I know, I know, you can't squeeze avocados online, but you also can't be tempted by the scent of fresh bread baking.
- Leave the kids at home unless you want to Plan-It-to-Gain-It.

Effective planning will reduce the need to go back to the store for a "few" missing ingredients. It's hard to resist going beyond those "few" and ending up with items in your basket that were not planned for and are probably not the healthiest. The main exception is fish, which is best bought the day you will cook it. (When you make a special trip to the market for fish, choose a basket versus a cart or walk to the market [if that's an option] versus driving to curtail your purchases. And don't let yourself be diverted to the cookie aisle on your way to the fish counter.)

Foodtrainers Menu Map

	SUNDAY	MONDAY	TUESDAY
BREAKFAST	R		
LUNCH			
SNACK			
DINNER			R
VICTORY LIST			

Shopping List

BREAKFAST ITEMS	LUNCH ITEMS	SNACKS ITEMS	DINNER ITEMS
Organic omega-3 eggs	Wild salmon	Pistachios	Chicken breast
2% Siggi's/ Greek yogurt	Tonnino's jarred tuna	Zing bars	Kale
Fresh berries	Mixed greens		Sweet potatoes

LBT Guide
R: Restaurant (check menu ahead)
T/O: Takeout

WEDNESDAY	THURSDAY	FRIDAY	SATURDAY
	T/O		
		T/O	R

LBT Truths

- ❏ Skinny starts Sunday.
- ❏ If it's not on the list, can't buy it.
- ❏ Plan for a green, a grain, and a main.

Strategic Staples

I am not going to bore you with 100 ingredients you need to have on hand. When I see those seemingly endless lists for pantry "staples" created by well-meaning nutritionists or chefs, I wonder how big they think the average person's pantry is—and who's going to go out and buy so much stuff "just in case."

To begin, chances are you probably have some "antique" ingredients in your cabinets or refrigerator. Purge anything if you don't recall when you bought it. It's better to have fewer fresh items you actually use than a lot of stuff taking up space. You'll be in great shape if you have the following:

1. **Hot sauce.** Eating just one meal that contains capsaicin (the compound that gives chili peppers their heat) reduces levels of ghrelin (remember that ghrelin makes you "growl," or increases hunger) and raises an appetite-suppressing hormone.
2. **Boxed (not canned) chicken or vegetable broth.** Boxed goods are BPA-free. Use broth as a base for soups or to poach chicken, or combine it with equal parts water for cooking grains to add flavor with minimal calories.
3. **Diced tomatoes.** I prefer boxed varieties such as Pomi over canned. Tomatoes are one of the foods where the antioxidant content is maximized when cooked.
4. **Fresh garlic and onions.** I cheat and get organic peeled garlic when I'm going to be doing a lot of cooking. A teaspoon of fresh garlic or ½ cup of

onions per day increases a key liver enzyme responsible for removing toxins from blood cells.

5. **Olive and coconut oils.** Look for extra virgin olive
oil, as this assumes the olives were cold pressed
versus being heated at high temperatures, where
quality can suffer. Coconut oil contains lauric acid,
the type of fat that helps you lose more body fat
when losing weight. It can also increase your good
(HDL) cholesterol. Try California Olive Ranch olive
oil and Jungle Products Virgin Coconut Oil.

6. **Spices.** Turmeric, cinnamon, and crushed red pepper flakes. Half a teaspoon of cinnamon sprinkled
on food helps keep blood sugar more stable. Turmeric is one of the most potent anti-inflammatory
foods, and red pepper flakes increase your metabolism in the same manner that chili peppers (in hot
sauce) do.

7. **Sea salt.** Most table salt is processed to remove
minerals and contains additives to prevent clump-
ing; it has nothing in common with the health-
promoting, mineral-rich salts we should all be
cooking with. I recommend using Himalayan sea
salt or Celtic Sea Salt.

8. **Good grains.** Look for black rice and quinoa. Black
rice has more antioxidants and fiber than blueber-
ries, and one cup of cooked quinoa has almost 10
grams of protein (bear in mind that a cup is often
greater than your "fist" size).

9. **Lentils.** Lentils, one of the best sources of "plant"
protein, are loaded with B vitamins and iron. They
do not require soaking, so they are much more con-
venient than other types of beans.

10. **Vinegar.** The acetic acid in vinegar decreases fat

accumulation and increases satiety. Avoid vinegar with added sugar or sweeteners. Apple cider vinegar and balsamic vinegar are two good choices.

STEP 3: PREP

Success starts on Sunday, but it doesn't demand a *whole* day of chopping and cooking. You can get very far with three items and one to two hours. In the recipe section, you'll see how a few ingredients can be used in different manners throughout the week. You don't need to subsist on these three items, but this is a great organizing formula. Prepping necessities include the following:

- A green (or green vegetable)
- A grain (or starchy vegetable)
- A main (aka protein)

A Green

For the "green" part, you may wash some dinosaur kale and wrap it in a kitchen towel to maintain freshness. If you're looking to branch out with kale, you'll find three different variations in the recipe section. Or maybe you steam two heads of broccoli or asparagus. And nothing is better, during the winter, than a tray of roasted Brussels sprouts.

A Grain

Boil up some quinoa using the Starter Quinoa recipe (see page 165). Quinoa can be used as side dish, in salads, and even for breakfast. If you're a rice eater, black rice is a nice versatile alternative to brown rice. Try cooking rice with green tea in place of water for an extra boost to your metabolism. And when you're roasting vegetables, bake a few small sweet potatoes at the same time to use throughout the week.

A Main

Grill a few chicken breasts, poach some salmon fillets, or prepare turkey burgers.

Prepping extra credit:

- Make containers of cut fruit or crudités (jicama, radishes, and fennel are more interesting choices, but carrots and celery are fine).
- Boil six omega-3 eggs.
- Brew a pitcher of iced green tea.

Cooking in Batches

I'm a big believer in making extra, but put whatever you don't expect to eat in containers immediately. You don't need two turkey burgers for dinner just because you have extra. Set aside the portions you'll have immediately, and put the rest away. I suggest dividing food into single-serving sizes and storing it in glass (Snapware) containers that are obesogen-free. These containers can be used for lunch or dinner the next day.

Whatever you won't finish within four days that can be frozen goes in the freezer. Be sure to use blank peel-back stickers to identify and date the container.

Promise

There's a fourth P in the Foodtrainers plan: Promise. The planning, purchase, and prep, along with the food suggestions, hold the real Promise of LBT.

Planning what to eat, buying the best products, and preparing them in the most nutritious and delicious way takes practice. Which greens do you enjoy the most? Are certain lunches more portable? If you didn't love a recipe the first time, maybe you tweak the seasoning to your own taste. Take notes and continue to experiment. Trust me: I have had many kitchen failures. Taste is personal, and cooking is where you make sure what you're eating suits you. You can expand beyond a green, a grain, and a main, but if you do nothing else, these three items will set you up very nicely. Whether it's arriving home from work hungry or wondering, "What's for dinner?" you now have the ability to divert many food booby traps and lose real weight. Instead of shelling out money for the latest supplement or cereal, the foods you purchase and prep hold real promise. You can now toss the Special K.

Five

The Witching Hour

'Twas midafternoon, when all through the workplace
All energy was gone without a trace;
The salads had been eaten at lunchtime with care,
In hopes that weight loss soon would be there;
Morning motivation now replaced with dread,
And visions of sugar danced in everyone's head.
—FOODTRAINERS LAMENT

"What is your worst time of day for overeating?"

I can't tell you how often I have heard from clients: *Everything is fine until late afternoon* or *I'm a different person after dinner.* At these times of day, your nutrition knowledge is irrelevant. Once your resolve has been challenged, it becomes so much harder to stick with your diet. Though it may feel like it, there's no supernatural creature suddenly dictating your food choices; you can control them if you learn to deal with your "witching hour." But willpower is not enough. You need to have your plan in place. Planning supersedes willpower. Once you conquer this trouble spot (not talking thighs or abs), real progress will be yours.

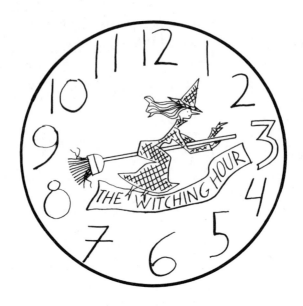

Everything's Fine Until 4 p.m.

Recently, I received the following comment on the Food-trainers blog (Foodtrainers.blogspot.com):

> *Do you have any tips for people who overeat between work and dinner? Because I have a . . . umm . . . friend who does this sometimes. And I . . . I mean . . . my friend . . . is having a hard time figuring out what kind of afternoon snack will hold her over so that she doesn't eat the caloric equivalent of an extra meal or two between 4:00 and 5:30.*

So many people can relate to this sentiment that my post responding to this "friend" is one of my most popular. Recently, I had a session with a client I hadn't seen in some time. This client is an Ivy League graduate. I mention this because I feel she approaches nutrition with diligence.

She's read everything nutrition related out there and has dabbled with many different eating approaches. And yet she came to my office for help.

I looked over her detailed food journal. Meals were perfect, hydration good, she was on an excellent vitamin regime, and yet something didn't fit. Her snacks were a bit of a free-for-all. I asked her about this and she replied, "I'm so good all day; in the afternoon I feel I should have a little treat." Hearing her own words, she smiled at me. We knew where to focus our efforts.

There's a reason for this insatiable late-afternoon snacking. According to the website Massive Health, the healthfulness of the food we eat decreases with each hour in the day. By midafternoon, blood sugar has dropped from lunch, morning caffeine has run its course, and the cravings commence. And if your eating throughout the day has been meager or inadequate (no breakfast protein, no "dunch"), everything can start to catch up to you.

For some of you, the witching hour temptation is sweet; for others, salty. Either way the hunt begins, you need your fix. Even the most dedicated dieters, who can be rock star eaters at breakfast and lunch, find that all bets are off come midafternoon. Sound familiar? What are you to do?

Sign a Pre-Snacktual Agreement

Recently I read an article in which the fashion designer Donna Karan referred to herself as a "uniform dresser" to describe the basic black outfits she favors. She's never at a loss for what to wear because her clothing choices are automatic. This concept can be applied to midafternoon food choices; your goal is to be a "uniform snacker."

A study from Dominican University found written

goals more effective than verbal promises. So at Foodtrainers we literally have midafternoon munchers sign on the dotted line. They pick two midafternoon snack choices for the week ahead and stick to them. We've found that once you're contractually obligated to your snack selections, you will take them more seriously. Use your Pre-Snacktual Agreement (page 53) or Menu Map (page 36) to make sure you have two clear choices for your afternoon snack.

For example, maybe one week your choices are veggies with one to two tablespoons of guacamole or kale chips. The next week you can select Greek yogurt or a nutrition bar. LBT snacks can still feel like a treat, but they need to be clearly defined. The fact is that *too many* choices can lead to too much eating. I scientifically refer to this as "pupu platter syndrome." You can conquer the midafternoon monster by limiting snack choices, writing your choices down, and honoring your Pre-Snacktual Agreement.

Afternoon Ammunition

In order to fight the witching hour forces, keep yourself "armed" for any situation: Like a healthy Easter egg hunt, stash snacks in your purse, your office drawer, your gym bag, the kids' backpacks, or the glove compartment. Finding those "hidden treasures" can save you from the unhealthy opposition.

Perhaps one of these snack snares sounds familiar:

It's 3:30 p.m. and you're picking up the kids at school. Lunch is a fading memory, and, of course, you have a couple of packs of Cheddar Bunnies "for the kids." You're starving and pop a few in your mouth—and then a few more. Most parents wouldn't think of showing up at school empty-handed; children need to eat. Well, what about you?

Pre-Snacktual Agreement

I, _____, hereby commit to my well-planned and love-handle-free future by preselecting my snack options. I am aware that the consequences of feeling in control and looking good in a bikini may include jealousy from peers and obnoxious comments from diet saboteurs, and I release Foodtrainers/Lauren Slayton from any and all liability.

My two Smart Snack selections for the week of __ /__ /__ are: (circle **2** Smart Snack options)

Feeling Nutty?	Feeling Crunchy?	Feeling Sweet?
40 pistachio nuts	1–2 Tbsp guacamole and carrots	Kind bar
12 walnut halves	1–2 Tbsp hummus and cucumber	Zing bar
15 pecan halves	Mary's Gone Crackers	22 Days bar
1/4 cup sunflower seeds	479° Popcorn pouch	Siggi's or Greek yogurt
1–2 Tbsp Barney Butter and apple	Kale chips	GoGo Squeez

This week I am committed to skipping: (circle **1** or more)
    a) Kid's snacks
    b) Office candy
    c) Munching while I cook
    d) All of the above

Signature _____

Date _____

Make bringing your snack just as second nature as bringing the house keys. The new checklist is: Keys? Wallet? Phone? Snack? Have reusable, adult-friendly snack bags filled and ready. You can do better than Bunnies.

Or maybe you're at work, trying to fend off your co-worker's candy bowl. Gummy bears aren't your favorite, but they're just sitting there and you're bored. Don't waste your energy blaming the candy pushers, who rarely eat the stuff but like people congregating near them. It's workplace bait, and you can only safeguard your snacking situation if you're armed with your own ammunition.

Snack snares are not isolated to weekdays; lazy weekend afternoons present their own problems. Your schedule isn't as organized and you may be home a little more. You can relax, but your Pre-Snacktual Agreement still stands.

Think about your snacking snares and anticipate them. Instead of feeling like they're your undoing, you can start to derive satisfaction from outwitting them.

Smart Snacking

Here is the LBT skinny on making Smart Snack choices:

- The best snacks have more than a few grams of protein or fiber, and ideally both. If you see zeros for both protein and fiber on the nutrition label, your snack is a zero. Pretzels and pita chips are zeros. Foods with protein and fiber will keep you alert and satiated.
- Smart Snacks should be 150 to 200 calories. If you're making the effort to be prepared, you don't want something that leaves you hungry an hour later.

- Space out your snacks. If you wait too long for a midafternoon snack, you will end up with the caloric equivalent of a meal. On the other hand, if it's 1 p.m. and lunch was at 12 and you're thinking about munching, it's not hunger. Smart Snacking is at least two hours after lunch but no more than four hours.

- Shun "container eating." Any snack can be abused if you sit yourself down in front of an ample amount. Divide large boxes into single-serving containers as soon as you get home from the store. This is a pound- and money-saving strategy that is often skipped. Don't skip it; we've told ourselves the "just one cookie" lie enough times.

- Or, if you can't be bothered divvying up, purchase single-serving sizes of good-brand snack foods (see my recommendations that follow). I'm not talking "100-calorie snack packs" or anything that screams diet food. ("Fat-free" foods are notorious for what the food manufacturers put into them to make up for what they've taken out.)

- Don't snack when you need a meal. If you waited too long for your post-lunch snack, have an early- bird dinner. If you need evidence, some nuts, a string cheese, a handful of "healthy" chips, carrots, and a few bites of dinner while you cook "dinner" is 450 calories.

Smart Snacks

- **Go for the crunch.** Chef Mario Batali claims that the use of the word *crispy* sells more food than any other adjective. John Allen, author of *The Omnivorous*

Mind: Our Evolving Relationship with Food, suggests that we eat crunchy foods for "the frisson of illicit pleasure they confer." Wow, so descriptive, and yet not all crunchy foods are "illicit." In fact, they can be stress relieving and satisfying. I recommend Mary's Gone, Orgran, or SnackMasters crackers; 479° Popcorn; and Food Should Taste Good chips. They are all LBT legal.

- **Nutty is good.** Raw nuts are a good go-to snack choice. My favorite nuts for weight loss are walnuts, pistachios, and pecans. Just be careful not to overnut. Overnutting is easy because one handful leads to another handful . . . Nuts are calorie dense because of their fat content (good fat, but still . . .). Portion out ¼ cup or 1 ounce (see the preceding tip on "container eating"). This translates to 12 walnut halves or 40 pistachios. Create your own "nut case" with a washed-out Altoid-style mint tin. Or invest in a few reusable snack bags such as those from Graze Organic.

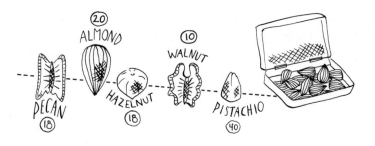

- **Choose "activity" foods.** Nuts in the shell, unpeeled shrimp, steamed artichokes . . . If you have to peel it, strip it, or otherwise make an effort to get to it, the activity serves as nutritional brakes and makes you more likely to eat less.

- **Seek out skinny seeds.** Seeds are often the forgotten sidekick to nuts. A study in the *American Journal of Clinical Nutrition* showed that the linoleic fat in sunflower seeds and hemp seeds decreased abdominal fat in participants by 6.2 percent without any other changes in diet or exercise. Sunflower seeds come in flavors ranging from cocoa mole to curry, so feel free to mix it up (just not on the same day). If you leave sunflower seeds in the shell, they become an "activity food." Pumpkin seeds, which are loaded with zinc, are an immune-boosting snack that works wonders for skin.
- **Nutrition bars** are preportioned, and the good ones are no longer glorified candy bars. If you're on the go, the nutrition bars I recommend are Zing, Kind (choose bars with less than 5 grams of sugar), 22 Days, and Health Warrior.
- Your snack should be a one-act play. Once you've had your nuts, seeds, crunch, or bar, that tired part of your brain may ask, "What's next?" If you want an encore, stick to vegetables: cut-up peppers, celery, jicama, grape tomatoes, or radishes. Or, if you have a salty tooth, try naturally fermented pickles or dried nori (a seaweed or "sea vegetable").

Snooze to Lose

Our bodies do best with a long sleep during the night and a short sleep during the day. What we mistake for hunger in the afternoon hours may actually be fatigue. According to Sara Mednick, author of *Take a Nap! Change Your Life*, in addition to promoting weight loss, napping can help im-

Best Foods for Sweet Cravers

I've mentioned a few healthy ways to satisfy sweet cravings, but wouldn't it be nice if you could actually decrease those cravings? Your brain may be telling you to seek out sweet, but there's another player in this sugar game and that's your "second brain," located in your gut. The term *probiotics* may have crossed your radar. Probiotics are bacteria that can help maintain the healthy balance of flora in the gut, often thought of as immune boosters. However, they may also impact your weight.

Researchers have found that the flora, or intestinal bacteria, are different in those who crave sugar versus those who do not. Other studies have concluded that obese people have different bacteria than average-weight people and these flora change when weight is lost. Interestingly, the gut is also where 95 percent of our serotonin is produced. Alterations or aberrations with good and bad bacteria have wide-reaching effects. Unlike Vegas, what happens in your gut doesn't stay there; it affects your whole body.

Fermented foods can increase these "good" bacteria and can enhance mood and reduce cravings. Additionally, the slightly sour taste may be another way fermented foods can help, as we tend to crave more of what we're eating. Sweet begets sweet, so less sweet just may lead to less sweet.

Try to include items from the following list in your daily diet:

Miso is a fermented soy product that's sold as a paste. Enzymes in miso prevent the growth of bad bacteria in the intestinal tract. When you purchase miso, choose miso made from brown rice versus barley. I like South River Miso Company and Miso Master. (Miso is an ingredient in Thin-I-Gette dressing, page 181.)

Kombucha is a cold, fermented tea that contains several types of good bacteria. The fermentation process produces acetic acid (also found in vinegar), which is a metabolism booster. I recommend Synergy brand; it comes in a good variety of flavors and has less sugar than others.

Pu-erh tea is made from the same plant as green tea, but it's fermented. This tea has been shown to decrease fatty acid synthesis and potentially lower cholesterol. It's mainly consumed as a hot beverage. Numi tea makes a variety of flavors.

Pickles made by a lactic acid fermentation process provide the probiotics missing from pickles made with vinegar. Naturally fermented pickles also avoid food dyes and artificial sweeteners.

Kefir, yogurt's healthier though lesser-known cousin, has a higher probiotic content. Yogurt is only required to have two types of good bacteria (called strains), while kefir has more than ten. Many people who are lactose intolerant or have trouble digesting milk products can often tolerate kefir.

Supplements may be a good alternative if you don't have access to fermented foods or want a backup plan. I'm a fan of the ReNew Life brand's Ultimate Flora. Regardless of brand, look for a number greater than 20 billion live cultures on the label.

Finally, I know what you're thinking when it comes to fermented products, but wine doesn't count. Even though it is fermented it's also pasteurized, which kills off all the good bacteria!

prove mood and performance, ramp up your sex life, and preserve your youthful looks. Interesting . . .

A nap of less than thirty minutes can do wonders. And there's a bonus if you have a cup of green tea before you head for the couch (or just put your head down on your desk): When you're ready to get back to your day, the little bit of caffeine is kicking in. And you've avoided the snack snare.

A short nap is also a noncaloric transition from work to home. It takes about the same time to kick off your shoes and have a quick lie-down as it does to rummage through the refrigerator to look for a snack. But many of us think that taking a short nap is a luxury and give in to many demands on our time. But if you think of it as a necessity, you'll schedule it into your day like any other health-supporting activity and save yourself all those "rummaging" calories.

After-Dinner Doozy: The Second Witching Hour

I often hear from clients, "I can be good all day but I'm a different person at night." One client's husband nicknamed her "Raccoon" for her after-dinner foraging habits—not the cutest pet name and not how we want to eat when we're trying to lose weight.

Research confirms that many people eat 40 to 50 percent of their daily calories at night. And eating at that time of day is rarely due to hunger. From dinner until bedtime is another of those transition times in the day that we often fill with food. Perhaps the kids are in bed or your work is done; now what? There is no metabolic need for calories after dinner. Despite the abundance of so-called healthy desserts, dessert shouldn't be daily. These pops and snacks are like methadone versus a full recovery. This is one of the behaviors that can change your weight forever; it's better to go cold turkey in the dessert department. Going half turkey (or Turkey Hill) doesn't work.

Alert: Those 300 calories from after-dinner snacks add up to 30 pounds in a year—probably the number you worked hard to burn at the gym today. And if you're thinking, "I don't have 300 calories," well, 100 calories = 10 pounds.

The Kitchen Is Closed

Is your heart racing? Does the idea of being dessertless terrify you? If you can't stand a day without dessert, have your approved desserty item midaft- 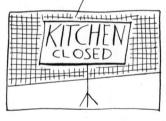 ernoon. Just as we did with the Pre-Snacktual Agreement for midafternoon snacks, make your postprandial plan formal too. Recruit a friend, spouse, or other family member. Most people have what I call a "candy confidant" or someone with whom you feel comfortable discussing food and weight. If you don't have such a person, anyone will do. In Overeaters Anonymous (OA), participants work with a sponsor. This support can be crucial when making changes with your food. I have new clients email me "The kitchen is closed" each night for two weeks when they start Foodtraining. Short of a refrigerator padlock, there's something about deciding and verbalizing that there is no more food today that's extremely helpful.

If a store is closed, you cannot purchase anything. *Kitchen closed* is just as firm. A Shape.com survey found

Timing Is Everything

It doesn't matter how late you eat, it's the calories in the entire day, right? Nope, sorry to say that's another of those weight-related rumors that can be filed under "Wouldn't that be nice" along with "A calorie is a calorie" and "Everything in moderation." When it comes to weight loss, *when* you eat may be as important as what you eat and is often overlooked.

A study recently published in the journal *Cell Metabolism* explained why. Researchers at the Salk Institute placed mice on different eating regimens for 100 days. One group, fed a high-fat, high-calorie diet, could eat their food whenever they wanted. Another group, fed the same food, was given only an eight-hour window to eat. The differences were staggering. The group with the unhealthy diet and no time restriction became obese and encountered a host of metabolic problems even though calories and fat were approximately the same as the eight-hour group. Furthermore, the time-restricted, high-calorie group was almost as lean as the control group eating regular food after 100 days. Not only was the time-limited group better off than the grazing group, they fared almost as well as those eating a healthier diet. Other studies have supported this concept.

Just as we've come to accept that sleep plays a role in metabolism, we may now need to realize that our metabolic pathways and digestive system need sleep or at least rest. In terms of putting this into practice, sixteen hours food-free is difficult (that would be 6 p.m. until 10 a.m.). *I suggest a minimum of twelve hours food-free.* If you finish dinner at 8 p.m., have breakfast at 8 a.m. the next morning. It's not only that we eat crappy food after dinner; it's that we shouldn't be eating at all.

---

that the encouragement received from sharing diet or workout details online motivates you to try even harder. Twitter just may make you thin. If you want my support, tweet me @Foodtrainers #closingthekitchen and I am happy to be your virtual candy confidant.

Think of it this way: We tend to relish whatever it is we view as the last hoorah in our food day. For too many people, this is their after-dinner snack. Many of my new clients report that they race through dinner so that they can get to their frozen pop or chocolate. If we don't have the sweets waiting for us, then we eat dinner differently. Your food day ends with dinner. Once you designate dinner as the endpoint, you'll enjoy it more.

A lot of after-dinner eating has to do with unwinding. Newsflash: There are other ways to unwind. Strategic sugar substitutes exist. I have a fortysomething client who purchased a Nintendo DS to occupy her after dinner; another pops in a meditation DVD. Knitting, reading *US Weekly* (the print equivalent of junk food, so indulge away), and taking up an instrument (Guitar Hero counts) are other ideas. And hey, maybe once you're not snacky you'll feel sexier and reignite "hunger" for your significant other. If "sugar substitutes" got you excited, sorry, but as you now know, no pink, blue, or yellow packets advocated here.

As you look for alternative outlets after dinner, beware of the television. Watching TV is associated with increased snacking and increased weight. Suzanne Higgs, a researcher from the University of Birmingham, has researched snacking and concluded that "focusing on the flavor and texture of food is one of the best ways to decrease snacking." The reason many of us eat more while watching television is that it impairs this focus. The same goes for emailing or talking on the phone while eating. When your focus is elsewhere, you will eat more and be less satisfied. If watching TV at night goes hand in hand with snacking, it can be difficult to decouple the two. Either make sure you eat without distractions or reduce TV time.

There is one exception to our after-dinner eats—tea. This superpowered beverage is completely LBT-approved for dessert. My favorite teas do double duty: They give you "something" to eat and drink, and they also relax you thanks to herbal ingredients. A British study estimated that 40 percent of tea drinkers use tea for psychological escape. Pukka has a Night Time tea with valerian and lavender, and Harney and Son's Mother's Boutique tea uses chamomile and orange peel. Check the label on your tea; even if it sounds mild, you need to see "caffeine free" spelled out. If you're especially antsy, branch out with loose tea leaves, an evening "activity food" if ever there was one. Loose tea tastes so good and there are some great tea producers out there. It's the thin person's nightcap.

Whatever you do, do not hang out in the kitchen after dinner to pay bills, work on the kids' homework, or use the computer. The closer the proximity to the pantry, fridge, or cupboards, the greater the hazard to your waistline. If possible, go to the bedroom or a room that isn't even in clear view of the kitchen. As a born and bred New Yorker, I know this gets dicey in small city apartments—"I'm *always* in close proximity to the kitchen," many clients say. In this case, closing a bedroom door or investing in a folding decorative screen can help. The sooner you can brush your teeth, the better. Speaking of teeth, adult braces might not be sexy but it's a fact that Invisalign and adult orthodontia can be anti-snacking weight loss tools. If your teeth are in good shape, disregard, but if you're toying with straightening or whitening, it just may have slimming side effects.

Wake Up Lean

At night, in the comfort of your home, it's easy to get sidetracked and morph into a raccoon. Rein yourself in by dangling a carrot or potential reward. *"If I say good night now, I'll wake up feeling wow."* Once you put an end to the after-dinner devouring hour, you'll sleep better, without too much food in your stomach, and wake up guilt-free and hungry for breakfast. So whether you are eating a full dinner before dinner or you find the raccoon relatable, you must plan for your trouble time. Only then will you be able to improve it.

Six

Treat Training

*My doctor told me I had to stop throwing intimate
dinners for four unless there are three other people.*
—ORSON WELLES

Everything Was Going Well Until . . .

You have a big presentation to give for work. You're well
prepared but are a little anxious about how it will go. You
picked out an outfit to wear and feel pretty good. After
all, you've been working out and eating well; you're trying.
The morning of your presentation you get to the conference room early. There's the usual unhealthy work meeting
fare: muffins, Danishes, and, of course, the plate of cookies
(your favorite). You remind yourself you're "being good"
and take a cup of already burned-tasting coffee as you re-
view your notes.

The presentation is well received and you're relieved. As
you leave the room you grab two chocolate chip cookies.
You deserve a treat, right? You eat the cookies on your way
back to the office. Once in your office, the mental scolding
begins: *How could I have just had those? I really blew it.
Why can't I avoid the sweets?* Pretty soon someone sticks
their head in and tells you there's pizza at the front desk.

You're in a bad mood. The day is already ruined and so you polish off three pieces.

This scenario is similar to stories I hear from clients almost daily. What went on here? Like many of us, this client felt that after getting through something difficult, she deserved a reward. In itself that isn't the problem. However, she wasn't able to eat the cookies guilt-free. She berated herself, which then perpetuated even more poor eating decisions. Most people can diet and they can lose weight too—until that first cookie or french fry. And then they are off. Their diets are "broken" and thrown into the diet recycling bin for possible use later. Guilt-ridden dieters tend to be less successful as they are trapped on the all-or-nothing weight loss (or gain) wheel.

Even if you are a *Little Book of Thin* poster child, you must learn what to do when you're thrown off course. Why not plan for those treats? Trust me; temptation *will* come your way.

I think one of the great myths of dieting is that you will get to the point where you no longer like unhealthy foods. There is truth to the fact that when you're eating better and exercising, vegetables, produce, and less sweet or salty foods will be more appealing, but if you're a cookie person, cheese person, french fry person, or all of the above, chances are you will always enjoy these foods. Whether or not you're trying to lose weight, let's all agree food should be enjoyed.

Many nutrition professionals have incorporated the concept of "cheat" days into their food plans. I'm not in favor of this; they're like a full-day food bender from which it is hard to recover. For many people, the word *cheat* is associated with feelings of guilt. I prefer to use the term *treat* for any nutritional dalliances because it's much better to focus on "treating" yourself—and following LBT strategies— so that you don't feel like cheating.

Treat Training

Once you have the Ten Steps to Svelte under your belt, have accepted your No's, and are selecting food based on the Cheat Sheet choices, when you reach the one-month mark—or when you feel you're on a roll with weight loss— it's time to work on Treat Training. At this point, you'll have the confidence to indulge. Mastering Treat Training may be the most important stepping-stone on your way to weight loss success. It will help you prove that French women aren't the only ones who can "stay thin." You too can live a balanced, Spanx-less life.

Becoming a Treat Master involves following four criteria, which help turn something guilt-ridden into something enjoyable, so that you can have your cake and weight loss too. You will be able to find a place (even if it's a small place) for special foods. Above all, you will learn the number one weight loss skill—regroup, regroup, and regroup.

1. TREATS, LIKE OTHER FOODS, SHOULD BE PLANNED

Often clients underestimate food situations. When we discuss social plans for the week ahead, I ask where they foresee challenges—such as when they go to a friend's house for dinner or attend a party. I grow concerned whenever I hear, "It'll be fine; I'm going to stick to my food plan." Then I ask specifics, such as, "What if your friend serves risotto?" or, "What about pie for dessert?" And suddenly they see things more realistically. For any situation, try to gain food information. It doesn't hurt to ask your host what she'll be serving, as long as you're not putting her in the awkward position of tailoring the menu to *your* diet. But once you know where the fat traps lie, it's possible to plan if or when you think you'll want a treat.

I promise that if you mentally decide to have pie ahead of time, you will feel very differently (and eat differently) than if you succumb to a pie surprise on the spot, feel defeated—and have a second slice.

So no matter the situation—a dinner party, a celebration, or anytime you are not in control of what's being served—try to *anticipate food challenges* and *envision the worst-case food scenario* so you can make it a best-case scenario. The correct plan isn't always to avoid all treats but rather to select the ones you feel are worthy and to keep them contained, which brings us to the second rule.

2. TREATS SHOULD BE PORTIONED: TWO COOKIES, NOT TEN

Before you get carried away thinking you've found a way to eat pie and pizza and still lose weight, there's a caveat. You have to eat quantities of treat foods like a person who is invested in feeling good. I have a friend who suddenly realized there was "extra" hanging over the back of her bra. She pointed to that "stuff" and asked her boyfriend, "What is this?" He lovingly replied, "It's bacon. Isn't that what you call fat on your back?" We had a good laugh, but you can channel your body angst positively. When treating yourself, stay connected to your own personal "bacon" (and your mission to lose it) rather than getting lost in the dining experience, disconnected from important goals.

You want to stay tied to your goals so that you don't get carried away. The best way to do that is to make sure that treats are contained and singular. This is a far cry from a full "cheat day."

I give clients some visuals to help them see what an appropriate-size treat looks like: the lipstick-size piece of cheese, a sliver of pie, or a fist of pasta. Additionally, it's not a treat *meal*, so there's not cheese and pie and pasta in one sitting (that's three treats), and there are no second "slivers" with Treat Training. This may sound harsh, but it has to be definitive before you start to eat. Along with mentally planning for treats, understanding the right portions is the best way to keep a check on things.

3. TREATS SHOULD BE CONSUMED SOCIALLY AND GUILT-FREE

While it's important to consider *when* you plan to have your treats, it's also key to know *where*. If at all possible, consume your treats socially (or in plain view of others). We eat and treat ourselves very differently when alone.

In one of her talks, Geneen Roth, who has written and lectured extensively on food and emotional eating, asked whether any of us would ever have a friend come over, have them stand next to us at the open refrigerator, and offer a little of this or a little of that for their meal. While I was always so tempted to try this for fun with a friend, I would never do it, and neither would you.

These eating free-for-alls are perilous when it comes to your weight and self-esteem. Brian Wansink, the author of one of my favorite books, *Mindless Eating: Why We Eat More Than We Think*, writes, "When people are alone, they may be more prone to have an 'eating bout,' which is a single episode where you eat three times more than you normally would. You're not paying attention, or there's no one else to give you social cues to stop eating, and you end up overdoing it." Call it a bout or a binge; if you can control where you have a treat, you'll be able to contain it.

Eating treats in a social situation also encourages you to

eat these foods for the right reason. It's very different having something delicious seated at a table of friends or family members as opposed to huddled in front of the fridge after a crappy work day or hunched over the counter because you're blue. You'll soon learn that a treat should be a positive experience, and Treat Training will help you get there.

4. NEXT MEAL OR SNACK ON TRACK

For many of us, once we've had a treat, our inner food and body critic may rear its nasty head and send us down a slippery slope. If this happens, take a deep breath and focus on your next meal or snack. This is how you regroup. When you plan your treat, consider your follow-up meal. Once your next meal is healthy, ding-dong, the guilt is gone.

As you can see, treats have less to do with the food we choose to have and more to do with the messages we send ourselves about our food. Self-compassion is a burgeoning area of psychological research with many applications to eating and weight. A recent *New York Times* story included a study conducted on female twentysomethings. The participants were told they were to be taste testers. Two groups were given doughnuts to sample—as much as they'd like. When they were done, one group was given a pep talk of sorts. This group was told not to worry about eating the doughnuts; everyone indulges from time to time. In the

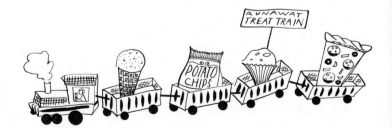

next part of the experiment the two groups were given candy.

What do you think happened? Sure enough, the group that had received the talk allaying their guilt consumed less candy.

Many otherwise compassionate people have low self-compassion scores. If we can learn to bolster ourselves, we avoid the runaway treat train. But it's up to you to stay on course. Remind yourself, *Two cookies won't do me in*. It's the head games and everything you eat subsequently that do.

Food habits and food guilt are hard to shift. If you try to treat yourself and end up feeling lousy, put Treat Training on the back burner, meaning no treats for a week. Some dieters may think it's virtuous to go without their favorite foods. And, granted, we cannot lose weight by giving in to every whim and craving. But as you try it, you'll see the value in mastering Treat Training, as self-reproach when straying occurs (and sooner or later it will) can be more costly than the most caloric food.

The Walkthrough

As with the "cookie" woman at the start of the chapter, so much of our thinking about food is retrospective. When we slip, we are inclined to say to ourselves: *Why did I eat that?* or *I didn't eat that well this week* or *I was stressed and didn't make the best choices*. There's nothing wrong with thinking about food. As the late (and so great) Nora Ephron said to *Gourmet* magazine, "I don't think any day is worth living without thinking about what you're going to eat next at all times." You can be food obsessed, happy, and thin as long as you keep it positive. One of the most important LBT secrets is reversing this process of obsessing about your mistakes and instead thinking about what you will eat in advance. Take control of your own food fate. Never make any eating decisions when you are tired, under pressure, or famished.

There's an enormously helpful exercise we do at Food-trainers called the Walkthrough. If the Menu Map provided a guide for your food shopping and cooking, the Walkthrough will inform your food decisions for the day. At the start of each day, while you're having your coffee or getting dressed, mentally walk yourself through the day ahead and plan your food.

If you're the listy type (love you listy ones), commit this plan to paper or type it into your phone, which immediately makes the plan more concrete. (I ask my planning-averse clients to email me their food plan for the day. You can get the same benefit by emailing the list to yourself.)

This anticipatory thinking has been used in other arenas. Charles Duhigg, in his book *The Power of Habit*, writes about Starbucks employees being trained to deal with certain types of customers. They practice what to do when a coffee customer is angry or aggressive so that employees don't act impulsively when put in a challenging situation. Duhigg also describes research conducted on patients following joint replacement surgery. Those who had written plans for their post-op exercise were significantly more likely to do their recommended rehab because, supposedly, they predicted where they would feel pain or struggle and knew what they would do when they encountered this. Doing the Walkthrough will enable you to see what the day ahead may hold, to anticipate food and related issues, and solve them beforehand.

Some food and related questions you may want to ask yourself:

- Do I have time to make breakfast at home, or do I need to pack it up and take it with me?
- Is there anything I need to defrost for dinner or prep before work?
- What about lunch? Perhaps you have access to a salad bar but maybe BYOP (Bring Your Own Protein) such as Tonnino tuna or Vital Choice salmon, especially if you're aiming for those four fish meals a week. Or maybe you're lucky enough to have leftovers to pack up . . .
- Do I need a snack for the afternoon? What was on this week's Pre-Snacktual Agreement?
- Any tea bags or Eboost?
- Will I need to make a stop at the market on my way home for any missing dinner ingredients from my Menu Map?
- Do I need to look at the restaurant menu online ahead of time if I am eating out? Will there be a treat?
- Do I need to communicate with my spouse, roommate, teenage children, or babysitter (each of these can make terrific sous chefs) about helping me plan and prepare?
- Do I need to place my vitamins near my toothbrush as a reminder to take them first thing?
- Are my gym clothes packed? Double-check: There's nothing fun about realizing your sports bra or a sneaker didn't make it into your bag.

In my opinion, this planning is more important than food journaling. It'll take you a couple of minutes but will save you many calories. More importantly, it will turn *Why*

Do-It-Yourself Treats

When you're eating better-quality food and feeling good, you may ask yourself why it would benefit you to eat some fried or sugary treat. One solution to this problem is to make your own treats and eat them with your family or bring them to a gathering. Try the Spicy Sweet Potato Fries (page 189) or Smart Avocado Brownies (page 190).

---

did I do that? into *I am so happy I thought about that*. Think about how accomplished you'll feel when you anticipate roadblocks and find ways around them.

I recently wrote a piece about guilt and eating. I was so pleased to read in the comments section so many accounts to the effect of *I used to struggle with food guilt* that ended with *but I feel so much less of it now*. Keep trying with Treat Training, because being able to answer your cravings in a reasonable way, without the mental noise, is one of the most important Plan-It-to-Lose-It tactics.

Seven

Family Style

*I come from a family where gravy
is considered a beverage.*
—ERMA BOMBECK

Marriage presents certain food challenges. Things get even trickier with parenthood, especially parenthood involving children between ages two and ten. Specific eating challenges need to be planned for. This advice pertains to aunts, uncles, grandparents, and babysitters too—if you spend time with children between these ages, I'm talking to you. In fact, some of these scenarios and the associated food snares are trickier if you're not used to them. When watching young children, adults are often sidetracked thinking about what the children are eating or not eating. Altruism has its downside. Many clients report that they were thinner before they had kids, and while children are a gift (some days more than others), they are a gift that will surround you with foods you don't want to eat as well as the present of baby weight that doesn't want to leave. Or maybe it's not even baby weight but toddler weight, middle school weight—the challenges keep on coming. It's best to prepare.

Birthday Parties

Think of how many kids are in your child's class. That's how many birthday parties (give or take a few) you'll be attending. That's also how many slices of cake you'll be offered. It's not an exaggeration that parents attend twenty or more birthday parties a year, per child, when children are young. Aside from the inconvenience and need to feign enthusiasm, there's the pizza, the soda, the cake, and the potential junk in the inappropriately named "goody" bag. Most parents are thoughtful (or simply healthy themselves) and put out a crudité platter. Consider that, and water, the adult food. Those are your food options. If this seems sad, remind yourself that most of the time these parties are at 10 a.m., 2 p.m., or other typically nonfood times. Chances are the children aren't even hungry, but that's another book.

Set an "I don't eat at a kid's birthday party" rule and practice saying "No, thank you" to the slice of pizza (200 calories) and the cake on the paper plate (250 calories). From earlier chapters you should know to have your ammunition or Smart Snack with you anyway. And for a caloric deterrent, do the math. If you have two children and

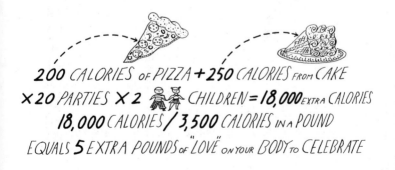

200 CALORIES OF PIZZA + 250 CALORIES FROM CAKE
× 20 PARTIES × 2 CHILDREN = 18,000 EXTRA CALORIES
18,000 CALORIES / 3,500 CALORIES IN A POUND
EQUALS 5 EXTRA POUNDS OF "LOVE" ON YOUR BODY TO CELEBRATE

do the above-mentioned party nibbling, you can gain up to 5 pounds a year from cold pizza and birthday cake alone. That's where good manners get you.

Dinnertime

Another particularly challenging zone for moms is dinnertime. Do you eat early with the children, or wait for your spouse, who gets home later? Many moms can end up eating almost two dinners. As I mentioned in Chapter 5, "The Witching Hour," *have the early dinner with the children*. Chances are you're hungry, and rather than pick your way through this time trying unsuccessfully not to eat, sit with your kids and eat. A study in the *Journal of Pediatrics* showed that mothers of young children consume over 350 more calories per day than childless women. A researcher on the study added, "368 calories could easily result from grazing on children's leftovers." No scavenging. Show yourself and your kids that you are taking a plate and eating the way you'd like them to. Nobody deserves waffle fragments, half a turkey meatball, and picked-over pasta destined for the garbage can. Other than being unappealing, these bites before you load the plate in the dishwasher do not register. Make a plate, with the foods you want to eat, and what the kids leave behind is their business. If you're inclined to compost, that's fine. Just don't give me "Waste not, want not." If you don't want food to be wasted, you may end up "wanting" to lose weight because of it. I'm happiest when I can eat dinner by 6 p.m. Indulge your inner senior citizen and give it a try.

Sit with your husband when he gets home, but do not eat again. If you think it sounds strange to sit with your spouse and not eat, your spouse probably will not. I had a client who said, "It's been a month since I've stopped eating with my husband and he hadn't commented, so I said something." When she pointed out her new strategy, her husband said, "I just thought you were paying more attention to my stories." This is the case for much of the food justification you do. I promise, nobody thinks or notices more about your eating than you do. This really applies to most food situations.

"Packing" Lunch

I am semigrateful my children attend a school where lunch is provided. I say *semi* because their school food isn't ideal; however, it still leaves me exempt from that annoying chore of packing a daily lunch for children. My boys used to attend a day camp for which they had to bring their lunch. I was never at peace, as I worried about whether our apartment contained the necessary ingredients for a wholesome, portable meal that didn't scream "My mother is a nutritionist" or "My mother didn't go grocery shopping." I realize that barely twentysomething camp counselors aren't rating campers' lunches, but as parents, we rate ourselves, and a subpar lunch sent out could ruin many of our days.

You know what else stinks about packing lunch for kids? Sampling their goods at 10 p.m., 6 a.m., or whatever hour sandwiches are made in your house. You know you're not hungry and you know what Pirate's Booty tastes like, but the food is there, most likely semiappealing, and so you have a cube of cheese or bread crust. *Make lunches after you have brushed your teeth, and see the advice for picks of kids' food that follows.*

Baking

At least once a week, if not more, a melancholy client comes in for a session. Their first words are "I baked cupcakes for my daughter's birthday and had to try them," or "The kids wanted to bake cookies." If it's not a birthday, you can cook many things with your children that don't involve sprinkles or chocolate chips. It's a blast (and sometimes messy or frustrating) cooking with children, but they are really just as happy peeling carrots or forming meatballs as they are making sweets. This is a great way to encourage children to try new foods and learn about healthy eating. I don't know if it was for my parents' selfish purposes, but I recall receiving a small omelet pan for I think my eighth birthday. *Given the choice, choose to cook something healthful with your children (but don't present them with a choice).*

I'm not suggesting you steam broccoli and take it to your child's kindergarten class for a snack. If you want to make a birthday cake or brownies, be my guest. Just watch

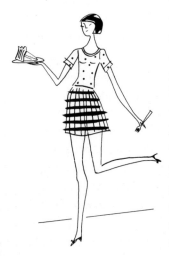

those leftovers. The brownies go to school, where they should remain. Don't bring home the uneaten desserts "for the kids." As for needing to taste what you're bringing "just in case," that's what your little taste testers are for. I know of one client who insists on taste-testing to be sure food isn't poisoned. Guess what? It's never going to be poisoned. When has cookie dough or brownie batter ever tasted poorly? Catch yourself; there are many things we can blame our children for (just ask my hair colorist), but we have to be adult enough to know that if we eat brownies we have to face the "dark" consequences.

Game Day (Can Be Almost Every Day)

Just about the time your kids are finished with the birthday party circuit, they're old enough for team sports. Sports teach children important life lessons and encourage time spent outdoors away from screens. Few things are better. I have two sons who haven't picked a sport or two as their favorite, so we have soccer, hockey, tennis, skiing, and baseball all in the rotation, depending on the season. (And a lot of sports are now happening year-round.) This is all wonderful except for the fact that every game, no matter if it's at 7 a.m. (gotta love youth hockey) or 4 p.m. (and thus ends at dinnertime) is followed by snacks.

When I grew up, there was team pizza at the end of the entire season or maybe a Friendly's Fribble (like a milk-shake, in case you're curious) when returning from sports at summer camp, but it's astounding that children can be offered Munchkins multiple times per week. And you can be sure there's plenty for parents to have some and usually one family bringing the extra twenty servings or so home. While I'm not here to talk kids' snacks, I do know that sitting in the bleachers watching a game (or texting and tweeting) isn't a calorie burner. If you are in charge of snacks, take advantage of great companies such as Peeled, GoGo Squeez, and Trader Joe's, which make snacks that have nutritional value yet will not embarrass your kids. And for festive fruit, try melon balls on skewers, clementines, and strawberries. And watch all that sitting; pacing the sidelines is strategic and makes you look really interested too.

Kids' Menus

A *lot* of my clients with children know what they "should" order and often do. They have the salmon or the salad. The problem is that there are fries or chicken fingers in close proximity on their children's plates.

1. TRY ONE WEEK WITH NO "PICKS" OF KIDS' FOOD

This is eye-opening for many parents, as the number of tastes and bites they usually take is way more than they thought. If you want to take this one step further, for one week collect the bites you would normally have and stick them in a sealed bag or container. At the end of the week you'll have a revolting reason why your jeans may not be fitting correctly—or maybe at the end of the week they will.

2. REMEMBER TREAT TRAINING

Rather than eating three fries multiple times each week, pick the one treat you are looking forward to and plan for it. And be a food snob. You don't want to waste your treat on average items. It has to be the best version of a particular food. This one treat adds up to fewer calories than all the bites and picks. Watch those three fries; other than children's feigned tooth brushing, they're one of the most deceptive areas of parenting. It's not the olive oil on your vegetables; it's the bites and picks that don't even register, except when they do.

3. CONSIDER WHAT YOUR KIDS ARE EATING

Kids' menus should be called "what your kids (and you) shouldn't eat." Selections are generally fried and nutritionally void, and your kids deserve better. Try sharing an entrée with your children or ordering them real food and taking some home if need be.

For me, as a parent my food-related hope for my children is that they grow up to be good, broad eaters. You need to realize that this notion of separate "kid food" and adult food prevents healthy, varied eating for both the children and you. We're so concerned that our kids will be treat-deprived or that we'll create "issues" that we often overindulge and oversugar our children. When I give seminars and talks, children are the most receptive audience. You don't have to hide your healthfulness from them. While it may not be for the end goal of thinness, children enjoy recipe and menu planning too.

Eight

Restaurant "Reservations"

A great way for you to lose weight is to eat naked in front of a mirror. Restaurants will almost always throw you out before you can eat too much.

—FRANK VARANO

My clients eat out. Many of them are out two or more nights a week, and often on the nights they are at home, they order takeout. It's my responsibility to figure out a way for them to lose weight despite these restaurant meals. They aren't going to turn down a work dinner, Moms' Night Out, or a date for weight loss. If you are working at things, exercising, and eating some meals at home, eating out anywhere will be okay if you follow a few simple strategies.

Game Plan

LOOK AT THE MENU ONLINE

Spontaneity in certain instances is good, but spontaneity is a problem when it comes to weight loss. Spontaneity, impulsivity, and "Ooh, that looks or smells so good, I have to have it" are the antithesis of *The Little Book of Thin*. Most restaurants have their menus online, or you can consult sites such as MenuPages. Hooray for technology! You don't gain weight perusing, and you can sanely develop a plan. My clients forward me the menus for where they will be eating and we make choices together. As you scan the selections, be aware of what dishes come with and order accordingly. Why opt for a bunless burger only to eat two cups of greasy fries? Do not be shy; "Can you hold the fries?" is all it takes. *Many pounds are gained and lost with side dishes.*

PRE-EAT

This may seem counterintuitive, but thirty to sixty minutes before your reservation time you want to put a little something in your system. The part of you that wants to hold off will probably eat with abandon at the restaurant, so "pre-eat" a little. Your pre-eating snack can be organic string cheese, asparagus spears, or ten walnut halves. You want to eat just enough so you don't arrive too hungry and, more importantly, you want to eat before you drink. As little as two ounces of alcohol on an empty stomach lowers your blood sugar at around the same time the bread basket appears. And alcohol interferes with the hormones that usually correct low blood sugar. If you're curious about the asparagus suggestion, asparagus helps your body metabolize alcohol. *Those 100 or so "pre-eaten" calories can save you hundreds.* Pre-eating will also help you follow that game plan you made.

GO FISH/BE GLUTTONOUS WITH GREENS

Some of my clients feel a bit iffy about cooking fish at home (until they try No-Fuss Fish), which means eating out is a prime fish opportunity. If you want to streamline your restaurant decisions, first narrow it down to the fish offerings.

You also want to look for a vegetable component if your selected dish doesn't include one. If you see things on a menu, don't shy away from making your own combinations. Mix and match one entrée with another's accompaniments. As long as special requests are made politely, they are usually honored. Chances are that fish you're now eyeing comes with spinach and roasted potatoes or some similar "green and white" combination. Your best bet when it comes to special requests is "Can I have double vegetables, please?"

DON'T GO FOR A FIRST-PLACE FINISH—OR FINISH-IT-ALL

When you're out to eat, are you the first person done? Fast eaters often eat more than they need to, and so it's no surprise that fast eaters tend to be heavier. You want to be the slowpoke at the table. Talk more, put the fork down, and try to be the last one to finish. Speaking of finishing, restaurant portions are gigantic. I am not sure when he became a health expert but I heard an interview of chef Bobby Flay ("Bobby Flay Fit" is a video series on Foodnetwork .com), who knows a thing or two about restaurants, and he said he used to finish whatever he ordered but now leaves something behind. Plus, he added, if it's not great, "I don't eat it." I say be thrifty as well as thin—only eat three-quarters of your food and take leftovers home for another meal. Another option is to recruit someone to share an entrée with you; if this sounds skimpy, I assure you I do it all the time with my husband (a grown man) and it's plenty.

RULE OF 1 OF 4, AND NO MORE

This is the restaurant rule my clients adore and use often. I'll explain. The four delicious problem areas when eating out are as follows:

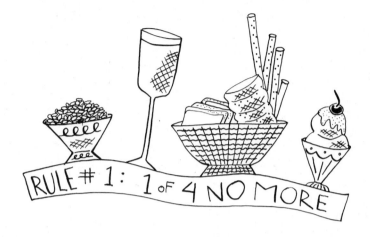

1. Bread
2. Booze
3. Dinner Carb (rice, potatoes)
4. Dessert

Bread "crusts," a glass too many of wine, some buttery potatoes, and "tastes" of dessert are "muffin top" producing. One client's husband said to her, "C'mon, half a cookie will not kill you." Of course it will not kill you, but it's those instances added up that can make all the difference.

Pick your pleasure: grainy bread (I know your local eatery is probably not serving sprouted bread—it's not ideal) *or* a drink *or* an approved "brown" carb *or* two forkfuls of dessert (if it's a special occasion and you want it to be your treat). Choose your 1 strategically. If you're with jolly, drinking friends, go with the booze. If it's sushi, maybe you know you'll be rice-ing. Perhaps if it's a birthday meal you'll leave the door open for dessert for your weekly treat. Whatever your selection is, you're having that 1 and forgoing the others for that night. Another night, another 1 of the 4. Got it? And whenever you can, not to sound like a broken "nutritionist," but make your selection ahead of time.

I'm Having _____ Tonight; What Should I Order?

Each cuisine has its nutritional standouts and snafus, items to pick and others to skip. Indian food, Mexican food, and sushi are the types of fare I'm most often asked about.

INDIAN FOOD

Indian food is mainly a carb challenge with delicious breads and rice; it's even more tempting to overcarb because of all the amazing sauces. If you're having a carb at an Indian restaurant, choose roti (sort of like whole wheat naan) or one "fist" of rice but not both. Select items cooked in the tandoor oven. Tandoori salmon, shrimp, and chicken are "thin" selections. These will be flavorful but less caloric as there's no sauce (less sauce = less carbs to soak up sauce). For a vegetable, cauliflower, okra, and spinach are good choices. Indian food is usually shared, so watch your portions; it's heavier food.

MEXICAN FOOD

The good thing about Mexican food is that most of the challenges come right up front. If you can get past the chips, guac, and drink hurdles, you'll be fine. When it comes to the chips, ask yourself whether you eat potato chips or other chips as snacks. If you don't, why would you eat fried chips, glistening with oil, before eating a whole dinner? I know they're really good, but ask your server for veggies to dip. Take two tablespoons of guacamole and as much salsa as you'd like, on a side plate, and dip away with celery or whatever they give you. As far as beverages, margaritas are sweet and sangria isn't much better. Worst of all, they often come in pitchers. Have good tequila on the rocks with limes or a glass of white wine if you want booze to be your 1 of 4. For an entrée, tortilla-less fajitas or a fish dish are tactical choices.

SUSHI

Sushi is a little misleading. Fish, salad, small little bites, what could be bad? For starters, there's more rice than you think crammed into a sushi roll; second, when a food has a "health halo" around it, it's easy to go overboard. One six-piece maki roll is plenty of rice if you're trying to lose weight. That one roll is equivalent to five pieces of bread or 2½ cups of cooked oatmeal. Stick to one roll with rice; most Japanese restaurants can make that roll with brown rice. If that sounds scant, supplement with a naruto roll, where the fillings are rolled in cucumber; a hand roll (cone shaped) ordered with "no rice"; or additional pieces of sashimi. You'll want to get a salad or steamed vegetables, or look for shishito peppers, which are popping up on sushi menus. They're spicy and addictive.

SALADS

Ordering a salad is not automatically a thin decision. Salads have their own clear do's and don'ts, and if you're eating salad in a restaurant there are a few things to consider. First, given a choice, you want darker greens. Spinach, kale, arugula, and microgreen salads are good choices. Way too many people think they are eating adequate veggies via romaine lettuce, cucumber slices, and tomato (the last two are technically fruits). As I mentioned in the Cheat Sheet, the real key to managing salads is dealing with what I call accessories. Avocado, cheese, nuts, seeds, olives, dried

Best Soy? Worst Soy? Should You Eat Soy?

I received the following comment on the Foodtrainers blog: "Soy—is it good or bad? How much is okay? Is the amount different for men and women?" I think soy is one of those foods that really confuse people. Since many Asian cuisines involve soy, here are my two cents:

To let the "soy" cat out of the bag, I don't think soy is the wonder substance or cure-all it has been made out to be. The way we eat soy in this country bastardizes how soy is traditionally eaten. For starters, there are some forms of soy you should avoid. Textured vegetable protein (TVP), soy protein isolates, and soy protein concentrates are shoddy, inferior examples of soy. Read your labels and skip foods that contain them. Additionally, do a pantry, fridge, and freezer check and toss foods made with these ingredients. Soy protein powder, protein bars, and faux meats and veggie burgers served by restaurants commonly use soy isolates and TVP.

The manufacturing of soy protein isolates and TVP requires heavy machinery and potent chemicals and leaves behind the fiber and many nutrients found in the original soybean. Think of bathing in toxic bath oil; even once you dry yourself off, some residue remains.

The cancer connection for processed soy foods is stronger than for traditional whole soy. Components in soy called isoflavones are similar to human estrogen and may fuel certain types of cancer growth in cells with estrogen receptors. And what happens when you mess with these plant estrogens? Processed, mangled estrogen, carcinogens, neurotoxins? Say "No, thank you."

Fermented soy products are probably the best soy

foods to consume. Examples of these are miso (delicious), tempeh (counts as a carb), natto, and soy sauce (I suggest wheat-free versions). Fermentation increases the digestibility of soy, adds "good" bacteria, and reduces the plant estrogen content in soy foods. When we look at the typical Japanese diet, about half of soy consumption is from fermented soy and the other half is from tofu and dried soybeans. In China, soy consumption originated when it was discovered how to ferment soy. This is safe soy.

Very high soy consumption can affect testosterone, estrogen, and thyroid hormone levels as well as iron absorption. For this reason, anyone with a thyroid condition or trying to conceive should, in my opinion, absolutely skip soy that is unfermented. Women with breast cancer or at high risk for breast cancer should skip unfermented soy as well.

If you do buy tofu or edamame, look for organic or non-GMO tofu (organic is non-GMO). For a word on genetically modified organisms (GMOs), I spoke to my friend and colleague Ashley Koff, RD, who has lectured and written extensively on the subject. She said, "Do GMOs cause autoimmune disease? Intolerances or food allergies? Cancer? We don't know *yet*, but we do know that frequent exposure to items that aren't exactly what the body recognizes add up . . . and we are likely to learn that they are adding up *against* your body, your optimal health, and your weight."

Do not add tofu or edamame to your diet if it isn't there already; aside from the concerns mentioned here, they're not the greatest foods for weight loss. If you already eat these foods, stick to once a week max and count them as a carb (soybean).

cranberries, raisins, and bacon may not come to mind when you think of indulgences, but when we're talking salads they are.

You know the fashion rule to tone down accessories? Sane salads have only one accessory. If you're looking at a salad with goat cheese, pecans, and bacon, ask them to hold the cheese and bacon. I realize that accessories make salads fun; I'm not saying no more fun, just organized fun. For the dressing, I don't have that much confidence that "on the side" will solve your problems. If you finish the dressing "on the side," it may as well have been on the salad. Ask for oil and vinegar or oil and fresh lemon wedges and use 1 tablespoon of oil maximum.

BE CHOOSY WHEN YOU'RE BOOZY

If you're like my clients (and those of us at Foodtrainers), it's unrealistic to think you're not going to drink . . . ever. If you don't drink, keep it that way. I've had nondrinking clients start drinking red wine for the antioxidants, and that's not strategic. We can get antioxidants elsewhere. If happy hour makes you happy or you like to have a drink when out to dinner, it's important to know what your drink order should be.

For starters, let's get the skips out of the way. Most of you know that when you're having piña coladas, frozen margaritas, and mudslides (so good but sooo bad), you've left the healthy reservation. Umbrella drinks are pretty much dessert in a glass. But there are some wolves in sheep's clothing being served up at bars everywhere. Take tonic; perhaps because it's clear, you may think a gin and tonic is a good choice. Coloring aside, tonic is very similar calorically to Coke. If you're not a Coke drinker, hold the tonic. If you switch tonic to seltzer for four drinks per week, you're saving hundreds of calories and over 12 teaspoons of sugar.

Martini glasses can also confuse. Unless you make it yourself, assume that ginger martinis, pomegranate martinis, and the good old Cosmo have too much juice or syrup in them, so they're "skips" too. Maybe this is a buzzkill, but knowledge is power (or inches in this case). And a word about glassware. It's ironic to mention this in a boozy discussion, but with a glass "straight" is best. Research has shown there's a huge difference (60 percent) in drinking speed between those who use curved and straight glasses. One hypothesis is that it's more difficult to judge the amount consumed with a curved glass. My conclusion? Straight it is.

In terms of glass contents, if you really want to be choosy, it's red wine, white wine, sparkling wine in a non-wine glass, sake (very low calorie, seek it out), or vodka, tequila, bourbon, or scotch "on the rocks" or with soda (as in seltzer). Garnish away with lemon, lime, or orange slices; even olives are totally fine. If you're an alcohol overachiever and want to know what the Foodtrainers favorite drink for weight loss is, it's vodka. A single jigger (1½ ounces) of vodka is going to run you 100-ish calories. Your wine? Red wine will be about 150 to 160 calories (wineglasses are bigger than they used to be). Plus, remember sweet begets sweet. I've found that clients are more tempted by dessert when they've had wine. Voli vodka is lower in calories than other vodkas and comes in interesting flavors. There's also a spirit called VeeV, available at most bars, that's made from the superfruit acai. If you're not a hard-alcohol kind of person, the best red to drink is pinot noir and the best white is sauvignon blanc, though wines, if not dessert wines, are fairly similar nutritionally. Cheers.

Nutritional Harassment: Is Your Boss Making You Fat?

Now you have confidence that you can pick healthy items from a menu—but eating well gets a little harder if you are not the one doing the picking. Things enter especially dicey territory when the orderer is your boss. Too many required dinners with schmoozing and boozing and that six-pack (if you were lucky enough to start out with one) transforms into "work weight." Often it can feel as though there are two choices—keeping healthy or keeping things harmonious—but I don't feel it has to be one or the other. So what do you do if your boss suggests a steak lunch or pizza for "the team"?

Supplement versus squabbling: There are times when "I don't eat pizza" isn't going to be well received. Suggest a healthy addition—for example, "Can we order a green salad with the pizza?" Chances are others will partake once it's there and may have been too nervous to say anything. Once the food arrives you can have salad and a little pizza or just salad if you so choose.

People pay attention to what you order, not what you eat (for the most part): When your boss invites you for a glass of wine or steak lunch, sometimes you can "go along" and if you're not interested in what's in front of you, you can control calories by sipping or nibbling rather than finishing.

Emily Post could order what she wanted: Flattery may just get you somewhere. "That looks amazing, but I'm going to try the fish" or "Thank you so much for the invitation, but I need to get some work done."

Doctor's orders: Whether it's reflux or cholesterol, if someone tries to steamroll you into eating steak, you can push back with "I'm not allowed to eat short ribs with my cholesterol." At times little white lies are better than lots of white food.

If these strategies sound a little manipulative, think about how manipulated you feel when you attend a business meal and are coerced into eating or drinking things you don't want to. With some forethought, "promotion pudge" is avoidable. And kudos to the bosses out there encouraging employees to exercise and eat well. That's a good use of power.

TAKEOUT

Although the general cuisine-related rules we've discussed apply, takeout meals are different because you're eating them at home. As we mentioned in Treat Training, our eating style can be different when we're out in public versus at home, often alone.

Takeout is often the last resort. You're short on time or have nothing that can be combined to make something dinner-ish, and so you place your order and you know what happens next? All of those random nondinner items get grazed on for those thirty, forty-five, or even sixty minutes until the delivery arrives. When your doorbell rings, you hardly need dinner.

Have the phone numbers for your favorite sushi, Thai, and rotisserie chicken delivery restaurants stored in your phone. Place the order when you're fifteen minutes away. By the time you get in the door, wash your hands, and change your clothes, your food will arrive. You may be tempted, but no nibbling while you wait.

Watch your portions; *don't overorder.* I know some places have minimum orders for delivery, and I know it's fun to try different dishes, but when was the last time you didn't have enough Chinese, Mexican, or other delivery food? Keep scratching your head, because chances are it has never happened. Most ethnic entrées are enough for at least two people. Add a vegetable or side salad and perhaps brown rice or a sweet potato and that's plenty. If you're ordering for one, stick to half an entrée, some vegetables, and a grain only if you haven't had one that day. Don't be afraid to augment with what you already have at home. Remember, you want vegetables at least the size of two Greek yogurt containers. Whether it's frozen organic vegetables or prewashed salad greens, this plainer component will make a delivery meal more balanced.

No eating out of the container. Do you drink from the carton of milk? I am going to guess you don't. Why? Because it's gross, and the germs from your mouth then find their way into that milk. If you don't (and from now on, you don't) plan on finishing a takeout container, don't eat straight from it. You want to visualize what you're eating so it can register. Take your sushi roll, salad, or steamed vegetables and combine them on a plate. Put any remaining food away. Use chopsticks to slow you down and don't even think of turning on the TV. This is *The Little Book of Thin*, remember?

You can absolutely lose weight even if a portion of your diet comes from restaurant or takeout meals. Having said that, you need some home-cooked meals in the equation. Even if you start with one home-cooked meal a week (and work your way up to four), that one time you'll have complete control over your portions and ingredients used; no "reservations" there.

Nine

Living Social

You Don't Have to Choose Between Social and Slim

My weaknesses have always been food and men—in that order.
—DOLLY PARTON

Many of us could lose weight if we lived in a box and made all our food decisions with no outside influence. That's no fun, but socializing does present distinct challenges when it comes to eating and weight loss that you may find intimidating. When you're making changes to your routine, you may wonder if it's worth going out for a date, party, girls' night out, or sporting event that could potentially jeopardize your amazing results. It is—because over time you will feel like social and slim are not worlds apart.

Having said this, I want you to be careful not to stack the social deck against yourself. One night out is fine, and even two isn't a problem, but if you're out more nights than you're home, you're going to feel as though you have less time to food shop, exercise, and sleep, and that will make losing weight harder than it needs to be. Keep this in mind when you make plans so that you have a balance of social and systematic that works for you.

Dating

There is an exchange from *Gone with the Wind* that a client always thinks about before going on a date. Scarlett is going to a barbecue. Mammy tells her that it's ladylike to eat like a bird in front of others, so she should eat a little something beforehand (pre-eating for other reasons). Scarlett makes the case that Ashley likes a girl with a hearty appetite but Mammy tells Scarlett he doesn't mean what he says. So Scarlett ends up having something before she goes on the date and mutters, "Why does a girl have to be so silly to catch a husband?"

My dating clients seem to fall into one of two categories. There are the Mammys who don't want to eat too much on dates; they want to appear dainty. On the surface, this restraint seems like a good approach for weight loss. However, if you swing too far this way and eat too little, you risk spending the night with Chips Ahoy when you get home—unless you spend the night . . . different topic. Then there are the Scarletts. Scarletts want to be seen as the chill girlfriend. Scarletts will have what he's having, whether it's steak, pizza, or dessert.

Why Fake It?

I understand there is posturing when it comes to dating, and this carries over into mealtime. However, there's going to come a time when your legs have stubble and you wear sweatpants. If you don't eat like a "bird" or a "hog," as Mammy put it, when left to your own devices, why fake it? If you don't intend to accept hair in the drain down the road from a guy, you definitely don't have to go with the flow and eat bread or grab a slice or a beer just because he does.

However, there is a difference between mindful and neurotic. Nobody wants to be known as the "diet chick" even if you are the diet chick. To avoid date weight, I have three suggestions.

First, make the most of your solo time and skip the liquor and carbs on the nights you are home. That way, if you're craving the pizza or the pasta he's eating, you have the option. You can plan for it as your weekly treat (don't forget the treat criteria). Bear in mind that snacks and alcohol are the two biggest contributors to love chub.

Second, cook for him. It seems like a caring gesture; it's a lot of fun to be in the kitchen with someone, but this isn't purely altruistic. Most importantly, the cook controls the menu, and if you want to keep it healthy that's your choice. If you're wondering what to make, try the Date-Night Salmon (page 187).

Third, men, though lacking in certain areas, get points for logic. Sometimes you need to connect the dots. Rather than "I don't eat pizza or any white carbs," which will have you instantly filed under "diet chick," you can explain, "It's important to me to look good, so I'll stick to this."

He wants you to look good too. A study out of Cornell showed men to be less tolerant of an overweight partner than women are. No matter how confusing and silly the dating world is, take some comfort in the fact that research shows that dating isn't nearly as bad for your weight as marriage or parenthood.

The Fridge Is the New Medicine Cabinet

Along with posturing, there's good old-fashioned snooping that's par for the dating course. Many people on dates and at parties flip open that medicine cabinet door, but I have a better idea: open the fridge. The fridge is the new medicine cabinet and will tell you a lot about someone's eating habits. If you spot a leafy green, yogurt, or any evidence of cooking, there's potential.

The first time I went to my husband's apartment, I spotted skim milk in the fridge and Ben and Jerry's low-fat Chocolate Fudge Brownie in the freezer. It was the 1990s, so his fat consciousness made more sense. As a nutritionist in training, I learned he was health conscious. More importantly, he liked chocolate. What more did I need to know? We've been married for fifteen years. The fridge is the window to the soul; don't let anyone tell you otherwise.

Converting

In new relationships, nutrition can be as much of an obstacle as religion. Carolyn Brown, a nutritionist at Foodtrainers, came into work one day looking forlorn. She had been dating someone and it was starting to get serious. I had heard he was witty and cute, but when I asked her how her date went the night before, she replied: "We went out to Five Napkin Burger; he ordered a cheeseburger and told them to hold the lettuce and tomato." He definitely

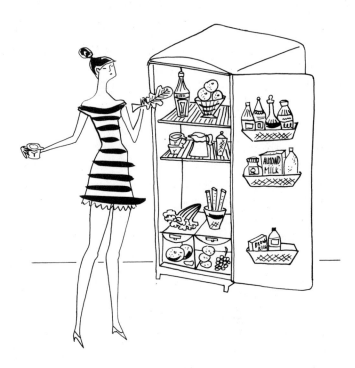

wasn't the "kale male" she was searching for; in her eyes it was all over.

Not everyone has an acceptable fridge or likes lettuce at first, so don't run for the healthy hills with the first instance of vegetable aversion. If things start to get serious, you don't need to initiate an eating overhaul. Start slowly; cook a healthy meal or go grocery shopping. People have been known to convert. And if you're looking to meet someone healthy, coed sports, food lectures, and cooking schools are good places to start.

I've also been hearing about a free dating site called SamePlate.com. SamePlate enables you to seek out potential matches based on food preferences. While I'm not sure a "diet dude" is any more appealing than a diet chick, food

The Ripa-Consuelos Theory of Salads and Sex

One day I was going into the office late and caught an episode of *Live with Regis and Kelly* (it was a while ago; no more Regis now). Bryant Gumbel was co-hosting, and he and Kelly were discussing a dinner party he had thrown. Apparently, Bryant had cooked a delicious and not-so-small meal including an entrée of Cornish hen. Bryant was lamenting that he made "too much food." Kelly smiled and shared a theory her husband, Mark, has. I'll paraphrase, but she said that when her husband sees her eating a salad for dinner, he gets a little excited, thinking there's a good chance he will get "lucky" later that night. On the other hand, if he sees her chowing down, he knows making love may very well be off the menu. Kelly explained to Bryant that when she devoured the hen she was served, her husband realized his odds later were not good. Brilliant theory. Of course, married life is different from single life, but health consciousness and portion control may have benefits beyond health.

likes and dislikes say a lot, so why not take them into consideration along with height and age?

Remember, *healthy isn't a turnoff, but high maintenance is.* On the other hand, you don't have to be the "chill" girlfriend because then you risk becoming the fat girlfriend and then sadly the ex-girlfriend.

Sports: Winning Plays for Game Day

I can hear the heckling now. Sure, the Super Bowl and the World Series come around only once a year. Though I'm nutrition obsessed, I know your "play" on any one day doesn't really change your weight or your health even if the Super Bowl is second only to Thanksgiving in terms of calories consumed. However, for sports fans, every day is game day, and socializing can mean enough sports food and drinks to ruin your season. I do find it ironic that some of the least healthy foods are consumed while you watch others play. If you look down and see a football where that six-pack could be, I'm talking to you. Try converting fumbles into MVP plays.

BEER

Any sports food conversation has to start with beer. I conducted a "scientific" study that involved polling a group of twentysomething guys and asking, "What are the beverages I should look into when writing about sports?" I came up with a one-item list.

Food Fumble: To burn off the amount of beer many people drink watching sports, you would have to play (and not watch) ninety minutes of football. And though I'm not suggesting you become a calorie fanatic, beer calories can easily range from 700 to 900. These are calories before any food. The biggest problem with stadium beer and stadium food is portions. One typical stadium beer is 20 ounces. That's really two drinks. Remember your budget? Four or fewer drinks for women, and seven or fewer for men. Sports fans, or those closely associated with sports fans, you need to factor in game day when planning your week.

Food MVP: I'm not a tremendous beer fan; for fewer

calories, go for light beer and stick to one (ladies) or two (men) maximum. Better yet, if you're tailgating or hosting, offer a drink that's less of a gluten fest. Bloody Marys are a great choice; they have a kick but aren't sweet and indulgent. Many stadiums have full bars or cocktail lounges. Yes, you may have to get up out of your seat to find them, but that's a good thing too.

SNACKS

You can't sit through a Super Bowl (or even watch Super Bowl commercials), a baseball game, or a basketball game without talking about snacks.

Food Fumble: One handful of Chex Mix or other snack mixes can pack 390 calories. I was shocked that a cereal-based mix could be this caloric until I saw recipes calling for a pound of butter. And don't even get me started on stadium popcorn or nachos. In addition to the snacks, so much sporty food revolves around condiments: the cheese, the sauce, and the dips. No food incorporates more of these than seven-layer dip, which can run you 500 calories in very little game time.

Food MVP: Pistachios or peanuts in their shell are a good choice. These are activity snacks once again; shelling slows you down. One handful or 1 ounce is 170 calories. Beware: Stadium peanuts are not sold by the handful. You need one or preferably two peanut partners or else I'll cry food foul. And when you go to a game and they check your purse, they are looking for weapons, not protein bars; it's not the airport. Don't be afraid to bring food with you. Finally, an MVP rule if ever there was one is: *Chip* or *dip*—but not both. If you are a proud member of team guacamole, remember that guac is good for you but bring veggies to the party and dip carrots, peppers, and celery. If you're one of those crunchy people I mentioned in Chapter 5, "The

Witching Hour," Beanitos and Way Better are top healthy scorers for team chip. If you must have it all, the chip and the dip, then your dip must be salsa. No questioning the calls.

HOT DOG OR HAMBURGER?

Food Fumble: I'm blowing my nutrition whistle and calling a time-out here. I'm not vegan or suggesting that you have to be in order to be healthy. I just can't cast my vote for the nitrate-laced hot dog or processed, worthless white buns. Frankly, I'd like to throw them both out of the game.

Food MVP: If you must "dine" at an arena, cut your losses and go bunless. Okay, we're doing better, and though, except in rare instances, that chicken isn't close to organic, I say chicken sandwich with lettuce and tomato. Lettuce becomes your "wrap"; add mustard (which contains turmeric, an anti-inflammatory—you'll need it) or hot sauce (a metabolism booster) and you've managed to do the food equivalent of getting on base under a lot of pressure, though you didn't necessarily hit a nutrition home run.

WINGS

When I say bucket, you think . . . wings! And if you think of wings for your sports menu, I say . . . think again.

Food Fumble: Two (yes, just two) wings with blue cheese dip contain 700 calories.

Food MVP: If you must wing, ditch the dip. And if you're home, serve grilled Buffalo-flavored chicken breasts or baked wings. That's a relatively tiny 150 calories per 5-ounce serving.

For some reason kebobs work well when watching sports or tailgating. The stick makes them a finger food, and it's easy to sneak in acceptably sporty vegetables such as onions and peppers.

* * *

I will admit, stadiums have come a long way. There's a gluten-free section and sushi at Madison Square Garden, and I've had soft fish tacos at baseball games. They're realizing that not everyone wants a footlong. Don't be afraid to buck tradition when you're making the menu or watching at home—Super Bowl Stew, Spicy Sweet Potato Fries, and Pesto Turkey Burgers all work well for sports spreads and lead to less of a postgame GI show (a losing play all the way). For recipes, see page 165.

Peer Pressure and Food Bullies

If you thought navigating a stadium healthfully was a steep challenge, try spending time with a group of women when you're trying to lose weight. My clients have unlimited access to email me. It turns out that many nutritional snags emerge on weekends. When we're out of our weekday routine, with friends or family or in this case surrounded by a bunch of belligerent bridesmaids at a bachelorette party weekend, situations arise. One Saturday, a client sent an email that many of us can relate to. She was with a group of women and was the only one trying to be healthy. Here's a taste of what happened when she passed on potato skins:

HEALTHY CLIENT: "No, thanks."

BITCHY BRIDESMAID (POINTING TO THE PLATE): "This area doesn't have bacon."

HEALTHY CLIENT: "No, thanks. I'm fine."

OTHER BITCHY BRIDESMAID: "Is it that you don't like bacon or can't have bacon? I would think there are a lot of worse things you can have than bacon."

HEALTHY CLIENT: "I don't like bacon."

ANOTHER BITCHY BRIDESMAID (IN AN EXTREMELY RUDE TONE): "I highly doubt you will BLOW up if you have ONE BITE, seriously?"

HEALTHY CLIENT: (shocked; I had no comment for that one, but almost cried)

Peer pressure certainly doesn't end in high school. It exists for adults, male and female, young and old, and can take many forms. Generally food-related peer pressure has less to do with not partaking of a certain food or drink than how your refusal of whatever it is makes the others feel. The key to food bullies is to understand that your declining what someone else is eating can stir up feelings of guilt for them. If you can take a deep breath and assuage their guilt, they will back off. For example: "Those look amazing, I'll try those in a bit." Or, "I had a lot to drink this week or I'd be drinking right along with you." Don't give your genuine reasons for forgoing; just make them feel better, whatever it takes. *Befriend the bully; it'll save you a lot of calories.*

Shared Fare

One of the most complicated food situations is when, as with the *Real Housewives*–like bridesmaids just described, food is shared. Small plates, tapas—call it what you like; sharing food seems festive and fun but is a nutritional nightmare. The person who suggests the food sharing usually elects himself or herself the meal director, and the fate of your weight rests in their hands. Crossing your fingers and hoping for the best isn't my kind of a plan. Short of refusing to share, here are some strategies:

- *Drunk driving is terrible, but drunk ordering isn't great either.* It's always a good idea to order with a sober head. Lots of things sound better after a cocktail. So make sure you get the order in before the drink(s) start flowing.
- *Place your moderate vote.* Even if it's unexciting, make sure among the dishes ordered there's a salad, side order of vegetables, or other plain item. If others do not eat these, more for you.
- *Keep track.* Whenever possible, serve yourself all your food on one plate so that you can get a visual of what you are eating and a sense of your portions. If food doesn't arrive at once, keep a mental tally of what you ate (one chicken satay, two summer rolls, etc.).
- *You are not a toddler and the days of having to try everything are over.* If it's fried, overly creamy, or simply not your thing, skip it.
- *Put on the brakes.* For some reason, food "for the table" is generally overordered. Take digestion breaks and assess your hunger. Stop when you're satisfied versus overly full. Ever leave a cocktail party assuming you would need dinner and realize you've had enough? One salad plate of food is really all you need. For the record, a cocktail party rule that may help you is "Two hors d'oeuvres, one drink, you've had more than you think."

In the same way that you probably know which of your friends to ask or never ask for fashion advice, you want to know the friends who tend to be food bullies or binge buddies. You don't necessarily have to end relationships with these people if they have other redeeming qualities. Instead, avoid setting yourself up for eating too much food you may not want and choose nonfood activities when making plans with the bullies.

Birthweek

I have a client who is pretty disciplined, and she was this way before ever stepping foot inside my office. Her issue was that she wanted to lose those pesky last 5 pounds. So we tweaked her eating, taking her from a nutrition B+ to an A–. She was losing weight and rarely strayed. I was confused, then, when during one visit I looked at her food journal and spotted more than a few dietary transgressions.

In this case, in a week's time carrot cake "tastes" were listed four times. I broached the topic of desserts, and the client dismissed me, saying, "Oh, it was my birthday." I asked which day was her actual birthday, and she said, "Well, it was my birthday week." She had gone out with a couple of different groups of friends, then with her family, and finally with her coworkers, all of whom knew that carrot cake was her favorite. Her birthday "present" in my office was 2 pounds to start her forty-fifth year. After our session, the birthday girl emailed me saying, "Oh man, the word is out; I better start telling people I love chia seeds instead."

I dissected kids' birthday parties earlier when discussing family time, but somehow the birthday buzz doesn't always fizzle as the years go by. Here's the thing: As grown-ups we really don't need cake and cupcakes to make things special, and we definitely don't need multiple pieces of cake when we're trying to lose weight. If you must, have your "cake" on your actual date of birth. For the other days in your "birthweek," it's fine to socialize and celebrate, but give those around you the heads-up that you don't need the cake.

And I don't know who started the rumor that it's bad luck not to taste the cake on someone else's birthday (probably the same person who decided that rain on your wedding day or a bird relieving itself on you is lucky). It's bad luck when you don't like the way your clothes fit. Once you realize all the instances where you thought you had to partake and show yourself another option, it's a real game changer (and weight changer).

Birthdays are one of those rituals we all go through out of habit, but if anyone wants to start the cupcake or birthday liberation, I'm here to help. In the comments section following a Valentine's Day blog post I wrote, one reader said, "If someone presented me with my favorite, healthy Green & Black's dark chocolate with ginger bar, I would embrace them and never let go." The truth is, whether it's a partner or a friend, those who care for you would be fine with candles in a fruit salad, bringing you chia seeds, or whatever silly, healthy preferences you have. So, if it's "your day," request away.

Beware of Brunch

I have no problem stereotyping—the female equivalent of weekend sports is brunch. Brunch, especially among those who are single or have older kids, is like the new weekend religion. Brunching is an activity and can be a rather problematic one when it comes to your weight. Many people have no issue selecting a salad from a lunch menu, but brunch—the combination of breakfast and lunch—almost forces you to choose something breakfast-y, which really means carb-y. Brunch conjures up images of Belgian waffles, scones, challah bread French toast, syrup, and jam. Brunch, even if consumed midday or later, tells you you're eating one meal where you would normally have two. And so clearly you are entitled to eat more, actually double. Brunch feels festive and invites drinking. And brunch usually replaces a Sunday workout. Great.

Whenever you can, think lunch instead of brunch. Lunch leaves you time for your morning workout and to have a healthy breakfast. Lunch is almost always savory versus sweet. If you're whining to yourself that you don't always want a salad, that's fine; go for eggs. You can have any style eggs, a cheeseless omelet, even eggs Benedict or eggs Florentine without the English muffin . . . with a salad on the side (you'll recall "Eat green, get lean" . . . if not, re-call now, please).

Ten

Are Your Workouts Working for You?

A twenty-minute walk that I do is better than
the four-mile run that I don't do.
—GRETCHEN RUBIN

If I had a dollar for every time someone told me, "I'm eating and exercising the same way I always have, but I am gaining weight," I could probably retire. Between ages twenty and sixty, a woman's resting metabolic rate (RMR) decreases by 5 percent every decade. Don't despair; there's hope. Even though exercise on its own is not the secret to thinness, exercise can help counter this age-related weight gain because much of that is related to a natural decline in muscle mass with age.

Exercise also helps your muscles remove sugar from your bloodstream. And despite what you may have heard, exercise reduces food cravings. Studies prove that morning exercisers show less brain stimulation when exposed to food photos than those who hadn't exercised. Brain activity, measured by EEG machine, reduced its response to food stimuli following forty-five minutes of exercise. And exercise can positively affect the hunger hormones leptin and ghrelin. Turns out you may not "work up an appetite" after all.

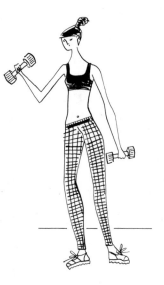

Workouts are a time to connect to your body and to de-stress. Plus there's a carryover effect: When you do something right in one piece of the health puzzle, you can channel that accomplishment into other areas.

I'm not a trainer or exercise professional. While I don't advise my clients on the number of reps to do, I counsel them on strategies to fit in exercise and suggest tweaks to be sure their workouts are still "working" for them. Seasoned exercisers have to take measures so that your body doesn't say, "Yeah, so what?" And if you are inclined to be a non-exerciser, let's figure out how to get you going.

Aggregate Exercise

Dieters are notoriously pessimistic, and what is viewed as a failure can leave us looking for the Exit sign. I give clients a number of minutes per week of exercise to strive for. Weekly goals allow you to miss a workout without panicking, and to make it up. It encourages "quickie" workouts versus waiting for "that extra hour in the day" (which, for many, only happens one day a year when the clock is reset for the end of Daylight Saving Time).

If you're not currently exercising—and you know who

you are—start with 100 minutes per week. The good thing about being a non-exerciser is that anything counts. Walking, dancing, and speed-cleaning your house can all work toward your 100-minute total. I love NYC trainer Amie Hoff's advice: Tell yourself you'll just do ten minutes (at the gym or for a run), and you'll always do more.

Every two weeks, add 20 minutes to your weekly total. Ultimately, your goal for weight loss should be 180 minutes of cardio a week. This is three one-hour or four 45-minute sweat sessions—or any other combination that gets you to 180. If you're a lifetime exerciser, 240 minutes or four hours a week is where you need to be. Yes, sadly it works against you that you've been active, as your body has acclimated to it.

You should feel proud of yourself as you start to fit exercise into your weekly routine, but just because you hit the gym doesn't mean you can chow down like you did when you were twenty (even if you could get away with it then).

Plan It, Do It

You set your alarm for 6:00 a.m. to allow enough time for a morning workout. Before you can shut it off, a thought surfaces: *Should I exercise today?* In that instant you are essentially asking yourself if you should get up out of your warm bed or go back to sleep. What outcome do you expect? This is like asking if you'd rather get your teeth cleaned or get a massage. If you hit the snooze button more times than the gym, here are a few tips to consider:

1. Schedule your exercise. Be specific! Don't just say that you'll exercise on Tuesday—plan a forty-minute run

for Tuesday at 6:30 a.m. Fitness blogger FitChickNYC has a feature called "Say It, Do It," where readers share their workout plan for the week. Planning and specificity are key.

2. Sign up for a pricey exercise class—financial accountability may ensure that you get there and get your money's worth.

3. Commit to meet up with a friend. There's nothing like a little social pressure to keep you motivated and on track.

4. Try to stick to the same exercise days and times each week and put them in your calendar so that your social plans are configured around your exercise.

You can reach your 180-minutes-a-week goal no matter what.

Variety Is the Spice of Exercise

Do you do the same exact workout every time you exercise? Are you wondering why it's not giving you results? Would you ever pay a trainer if they did identical workouts each time you showed up? Same exercise = same body.

While it's good to stick to the same exercise days every week, your routine should vary in terms of intensity and duration. Once you are working out enough and hitting your weekly budget, plan for one *intense* day in your week. Your intense workout is perfect for days when you are short on time, as this kind of session should be thirty-five minutes or less—but harder than your typical workout.

Additionally, pick one *long* day a week. People who have trained for a marathon or triathlon are accustomed to one

Foodtrainers Dream Exercise Week

	SUNDAY	MONDAY	TUESDAY	WEDNESDAY	THURSDAY	FRIDAY	SATURDAY	TOTAL CARDIO
NEWBIE EXECISER	Cardio (fast walk/ optional run) 30 min	Off	Cardio 35 min	Off	Off	Cardio 35 min	Off	100 min
MODERATE EXERCISER	Cardio 40 min	"Intense" day cardio 30 min	Cardio 40 min	Optional yoga/ strength	Cardio 40 min	Off	Long run/ bike 50+ min	180–200 min
LIFETIME EXERCISER	"Long" day cardio 60+ min	Cardio 45 min	Optional yoga/ strength	"Double-header" cardio 80+ min	Cardio 40 min	"Intense" day cardio 30 min	Off	>240 min

long run or ride a week. If your workouts are always thirty minutes, once a week move up to forty minutes or take a regular forty-five-minute workout to an hour.

The third way to spice up your exercise is with a *double header*. Though two games in a row is awful in baseball (I'm someone who thinks the seventh-inning "stretch" is where you stretch over to the parking lot and head home), two back-to-back sessions are good for your weight. Double-header workouts could be your own personal duathlon: a run followed by a bike ride or swim. It can also be done within the confines of a gym. Perhaps you will tack on some cardio before a spin class or start out on the rowing machine and follow it up with the stair climber (two brutal and underused pieces of exercise equipment).

Yoga and Emotional Eating

There's nothing like the stress release of a sweaty spin class or long run, but when it comes to emotional eating and bingeing, there are some interesting findings on the benefits of yoga. Depending on where you fall on the emotional eating spectrum (I'm convinced we're all on the spectrum somewhere), food can be used to escape certain thoughts or situations. It's sort of systemic Novocain. Yoga can counter these tendencies. Rather than being detached from our bodies, yoga gets us to focus on our bodies. Instead of escaping (via eating), yoga can keep us present. If you feel I'm getting New Agey, you could probably use a yoga class.

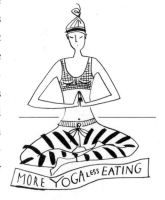

MORE YOGA LESS EATING

In one study, a twelve-week yoga program resulted in participants having fewer binge episodes, increased self-esteem, and decreased body mass index (BMI). And this program included only one yoga session a week. If you're looking for a tool to combat stress or "depressed" eating, yoga can help you immensely. (I'm sorry to report, however, that yoga minutes do not count toward your weekly cardio budget.)

Preworkout and Postworkout Snacks

I blame the popularity of marathons and triathlons for leading people to believe they need preworkout and post-workout snacks, even if they go for a thirty-minute walk. There's also the "I deserve" trap if you feel you are owed a snack or food reward in exchange for exertion. This compensation is really a booby prize (or maybe a bigger "booty" prize) that counteracts the advantages of exercise. It's important to remind yourself what your goal is.

When it comes to exercise, nutrition advice is different for sports performance versus weight loss.

1. If you work out first thing in the morning, I suggest working out "on empty," that is, before you eat anything. An Australian study found that exercising before eating led to higher levels of muscle protein, which helps glucose leave the bloodstream. Exercising in a fasted state compels your body to use more body fat for fuel.

2. Morning preworkout eating is discouraged; post-workout eating is another story. Exercise lowers your blood sugar, and if you wait too long following a workout, you will end up eating more calories than

you burned. Eat within thirty minutes of working out, and be sure to eat some protein. (My first choice for a protein snack is a Matcha Colada smoothie. See page 178 for this powdered green tea–based drink.) When that sabotaging part of your brain says, "I deserve a treat for my exertion," this is it. Another post-workout option, especially if it's later in the day, is eggs (muffin frittatas are portable and delicious). Try the LBT recipe for kale frittatas or, as we call them, Green Eggs (page 169).

Why Your Workout May Not Be Cutting It

There's a critical aspect of weight loss that I refer to as OTID: the Other Twenty-three hours In the Day. If you do a spin class each morning and then sit for the rest of the day, you are missing out on precious calorie-burning opportunities. Exercise is important, but so is activity. In fact, it may be more important, because research proves that as we sit, our bodies redirect fat toward storage—horrifying but true.

There's a popular misconception that if you get enough exercise, you're exempt from the negative consequences of sitting. Sorry to say, gym-going isn't your ticket to sit. What you do in your non-exercise hours can be the difference between you and those last 5 pounds.

There's a lot that you can do without having to change into workout gear:

1. Get off the bus or train one stop early.

2. Meet in person versus Skyping, teleconferencing, or emailing. Technology may be providing us all with more than convenience ("Techie tush"? No, thanks).

3. Stand while you work. At home, I put my laptop on the kitchen counter (which works perfectly unless I'm hungry). Use a balance ball for a desk chair. (Gaiam makes a balance ball chair with a small stand so you can work your muscles without tipping over.)

4. Two full water bottles make excellent hand weights you can use from the comfort of a work cubicle.

5. Take the stairs instead of the elevator.

6. Play with your kids instead of just watching them at play. (And make sure they are playing at something physical, not electronic.)

7. Do push-ups or crunches for the duration of TV commercials.

8. You can hide the remote, thus forcing you to stand up in order to change the channel—because none of us can stick to just one channel.

9. We've test-driven the Fitbit in our offices, and it's our favorite activity device. Fitbits, Nike FuelBands, and Jawbone UP Bands are the next-generation pedometers.

10. And finally, feel free to "spice it up." OTID is all about maximizing those other twenty-three hours. Anything counts, and your partner can thank us for this last suggestion.

Eleven

Trimming Your Travel

Healthy Itineraries

*It's not cheating when you're in a different
zip code or a different state.*
—*ROAD TRIP* MOVIE

One of my Foodtrainees—we'll call her JB—is a picture-perfect planner at home; she has her healthy system down pat. She's great with her daily Walkthrough, Menu Map, and cooking, and she always finds time for exercise. Home is predictable. But she travels a fair amount for work, and it really throws her. She seems like two different people— the organized, all-her-snacks-in-a-row home client and then systemless when away. Between time changes, erratic exercise, and insufficient sleep, JB (short for "jet blues") feels destined to eat poorly before she's even departed, which, of course, impacts her efforts. There's something about being far from home that can make weight loss goals feel distant or less pressing.

Fortunately for her, she's found a method for dealing with potentially maddening travel. She knows that a vacation mind-set doesn't work when you travel frequently, no matter how annoyed you are to be on the road (again). JB knows what food to bring and what obstacles to anticipate, and this has boosted her confidence. Rather than resenting the travel, she has organized it and made it work. The first time you show yourself you can solve a food snare, you no longer feel helpless. Success breeds success.

I suggest rereading this chapter before every trip.

Travel Insurance: Create a Food First-Aid Kit

I carried a first-aid kit around in the diaper bag everywhere we traveled for the first few years of my children's lives; many neurotic mothers do. When I used my Band-Aids or Neosporin, I felt like a gold star parent there at the ready with the necessary remedy. There were things in there like syrup of ipecac that went unused (thank goodness), but even these items served a purpose. They convinced me I was parentally prepared. A Food First-Aid Kit will show that you can go on a trip of any duration and handle any situation with your weight unscathed. *Every vacation temptation has its tonic.* Never utter "That's all that was there" again.

- *Jet lag:* Try Eboost, your powdered green tea (which also works nicely as a poolside "mocktail"). To help you sleep, Zyflamend PM contains valerian as well as anti-inflammatory ginger and turmeric.
- *Bloat or "plane puffies":* Drinking Yogi detox tea with cardamom, fennel, and other herbs or chewing on a pinch of fennel seeds will ensure that you get off the plane feeling the same.
- *Dreaded delays:* Do not stray; your nut case is there for a reason. Fill it with twelve omega-3-rich walnuts

(anti-inflammatory) or 3 tablespoons of pumpkin seeds (skin savers). Portion-controlled Barney Butter almond butter packs also do the trick.

- *Continental aka "carbinental" breakfast:* There's no reason to croissant, especially if you're in San Antonio or Salt Lake City versus Paris; bring a Blender Bottle and envelopes of protein powder and you can start your day on track.
- For those *sad, standard sandwich trays* at lunchtime, jerky has come a long way. I'm partial to the Slant-Shack brand.
- *Green juice withdrawal:* While I've pushed the envelope in terms of "travel items," you're not lugging your juicer with you. For juice fanatics, that can be disheartening. Have no fear; your morning methadone is here. Raw Reserve from Amazing Grass is your "travel greens."
- *Ski jacket snack:* Pack Zing or Health Warrior bars, and don't even think of justifying a baked good based on calories burned skiing. If you're not skiing, bars work well for any jacket or anytime you're confronted with a cookie plate.
- *Vacation constipation:* CocoChia can be very effective, though not too effective. If you don't have Coco-Chia (chia, coconut, and probiotic packs), plain chia seeds will do.
- *Tummy turbulence:* For food poisoning or even sniffles and non-GI ailments, take ReNew Life Probiotics at the first sign things aren't right.
- *Happier hour:* Snack on olives, especially Oloves brand's Hot Chili Mama flavor.
- *Minibar magnetism:* Resist the urge to be ripped off and sugared. Sweet Riot to the rescue: A few of these

Food First-Aid Kit Essentials

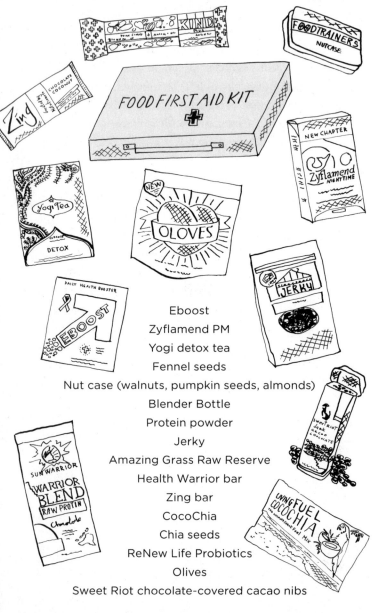

Eboost

Zyflamend PM

Yogi detox tea

Fennel seeds

Nut case (walnuts, pumpkin seeds, almonds)

Blender Bottle

Protein powder

Jerky

Amazing Grass Raw Reserve

Health Warrior bar

Zing bar

CocoChia

Chia seeds

ReNew Life Probiotics

Olives

Sweet Riot chocolate-covered cacao nibs

chocolate-covered cacao nibs will satisfy you. Sprinkle a few more over the walnuts in your nut case.

Check the contents of your Food First-Aid Kit before your departure; you may need to replenish your supplies from trip to trip. Eagle Creek, the packing wizards, makes packing cubes and half cubes that work perfectly for Food First-Aid Kits. Pick anything that zips shut and that's mesh or transparent so you can see the contents. You're worth more than a plastic zip-top bag, but in a pinch, that's fine.

Pre- and Post-Trip Strict

Travel eating involves more restaurant meals and more packaged or convenience foods and snacks. The day before *and* the day after getting home, eat only nonpackaged foods for twenty-four hours. I call these Whole Foods Days.

Whole Foods Day Sample Menu

Breakfast: Eggs and ½ avocado

Midmorning: Pu-erh tea, 16 ounces water right before lunch

Lunch: Arugula, kale, or microgreens salad with Starter Chicken Cutlets (page 171) or Essential Poached Salmon (page 186), cucumbers, radishes, and yellow peppers

Midafternoon: Pumpkin or sunflower seeds, 16 ounces water preceding dinner

Dinner: Shrimp and veggies

After Dinner: Herbal tea

ANCHOR AND FLEX

While your eating may not be picture-perfect on a trip, you need to stay centered. An Anchor Behavior is the one area you stick to without question. Whether it's Tuscany, Tel Aviv, or Turks and Caicos, wherever your travels take you, *think of the habits we've discussed and pick one to stick to consistently for the duration of your trip.* Can you keep breakfast on track (after all, there's plenty of time to play later)? Or maybe you'll hydrate and drink your tea? Perhaps you're finding dessert-doesn't-work to be productive; then that's your answer. You can't always do everything to the letter when away, but you want something that sends the message to your brain (and thighs) that you're connected to losing weight. You may be away but you bring your body with you, and you can bring it home in as good a shape as you when you left.

Now comes your Flex Area. I'm sorry to say we can't eat and drink anything and everything, sit on a beach chair, and lose weight. Wouldn't that be nice? I've seen this vacation fantasy thinking play out, and these clients end up in my office, living proof that the piña colada plan isn't a good one. You also want to make your Flex Area worth it. Don't waste calories on conference room standard fare (sandwiches, cookies—who decided this was the way to feed working people anyway?). When you pick your Flex Area, pick your pleasure—you can skip some workouts or imbibe or carb a bit more, within reason, but not all up the wazoo.

TRAVEL DAYS OR DAZE

Avoid airline food at all costs (if you are actually served anything).

I don't care if it's business class or coach. Our bodies

don't care if it's cheap or free. That applies to airline food, "goody" bags (or "not so goody" bags), gratis food at the hotel, you name it. On certain airlines the food may look decent or taste fine (doubtful), but it's still brimming with sodium and preservatives, not to mention bacteria. In terms of calories, the average airplane meal has 950 calories. Bring a salad, brown rice sushi, or a sandwich on sprouted bread instead (Starter Chicken Cutlets on Ezekiel bread with baby spinach and hummus works well). Also be aware that you don't need to eat in every time zone. On travel days, pick a clock and eat your meals on that schedule. You don't need to eat breakfast if it's really the middle of the night. This will not help you "adjust" or combat jet lag, I promise.

Airport food isn't fantastic, but it's not an absolute no-no. You'll have your Food First-Aid Kit, but if you're stuck in an airport for an extended period of time, you'll need to conjure up your detective skills. You are on a scavenger hunt for healthy items. Chances are you will not find everything from one purveyor. Maybe you'll get a green tea and fruit salad from Starbucks, steamed vegetables from Panda Express or a Mexican restaurant, and nuts from the newsstand.

DRINK (WATER)

It's very easy to get dehydrated when you travel, which actually leaves you more vulnerable to airborne germs, jet lag, and mindless munching. Bring your reusable nonplastic water bottle or a travel mug with you. Once you clear security you'll be able to fill it at a water fountain. When you're finally on board, use your tea bags; green tea, pu-erh tea (fermented tea), Yogi detox tea, and ginger tea are good options.

Road Rules

So you have the Whole Foods Day for before and after your trip, and your Food First-Aid Kit is stocked. What about the trip itself? It's one thing being loosey-goosey if you take only one trip a year. Even then, I am unconvinced that "eatingpalooza" type food behavior ever feels good for anyone who is weight or wellness conscious.

Two Nutritionists, the Denver Airport, and the Amazing Healthy Food Race

I was coming home from a nutrition conference with my friend and colleague Keri Glassman. We had cut it a little close with our timing before a flight and found ourselves with thirty minutes to sort out dinner in a food court. We always treat our business trips as a child-free opportunity to eat superclean and we were not going to be derailed. We probably looked like lunatics as we scurried off in opposite directions frantically reviewing our options. We ended up with a salad with black beans, avocado, and grilled vegetables. We had divided and conquered the healthy eating conundrum; I'd be lying if I said we weren't impressed with our own ingenuity. You too will find something to tide you over, and when you tame the airport beast or find decent options in a junky jungle, it's especially gratifying.

DRINKS

Often, when you are out every night, more nights out can encourage more drinking. However, if you have a couple of glasses of wine per night on a one-week trip, that's fourteen drinks (too many). Can you skip a night? Keep it to one drink on the others? If you do, you're down to six and may be able to break even on the scale, which is a weight success when it comes to travel. Doing the math is much more strategic than "I will not drink too much."

NO DAY DRINKING

Maybe I'm biased from the lovely city of drinkers I counsel every day, but vacation often means every hour is happy hour. This is dangerous. Lunch drinking makes you more likely to eat the wrong things, nap away your afternoon, and wake up just in time to drink again. Cocktails are fine at cocktail hour; just stick to your planned number.

EXERCISE

Exercise when away is a great way to stay connected to your healthy habits but requires troubleshooting. I love this quote from an article in the *Wall Street Journal*: "Thinking about going to the gym burns between 0 and 0 calories."

What time do you arrive and leave? Sometimes travel days are realistically out when scheduling a workout; however, if you are off from work those days with time to spare, nothing feels better than sneaking in exercise before getting on a plane.

What's on the agenda? What are your workout options? If you're sitting in a conference room all day, a good sweat beforehand can energize you. If that hotel gym is pretty dingy, don't despair; there's no better way to see a new city than going for a run. If nothing else, even fifteen minutes of planks, push-ups, triceps dips, and water-bottle biceps curls is better than nothing and can be done in any hotel room. Take advantage of fitness apps, a real savior when traveling. Nike Fitness has a great one that's like having a personal trainer with you.

Pick a number of minutes you can commit to. If a trip is less than forty-eight hours, you just need to pack and then use those workout clothes. For longer trips, if you can't get your full 180 or more weekly minutes in, aim for 150 minutes minimum for a one-week trip. Twenty minutes of exercise per day may keep travel weight gain at bay. Know yourself and decide what you can commit to. If you're going to be sightseeing for hours on end—lots of OTID (Other Twenty-three hours In the Day)—will you really get on the treadmill when you get back to the hotel?

ROAD WARRIOR CHECKLIST

Make sure you pack all the necessary items to encourage exercise: A jump rope, TRX bands, or something called the FitKit (a way to get in a strength workout anywhere) will eliminate every exercise excuse while you're away. A bunch of successful Foodtrainees bring a scale with them on vacation; it's not something I suggested but does produce good results. One client said, "Carrying that scale prevents coming home with unpleasant surprises."

DELAY YOUR PLAY

While your Cheat Sheet doesn't list scones, fettuccine, or naan, I understand wanting to taste the local fare when you travel. Maybe you're curious about Texas barbecue or have to have Chicago-style pizza. If the thought of forgoing a certain food is going to fill you with long-term regret, there's a way for you to have it. First, on your Glad Libs sheet (discussed shortly), think about your destination, and if there's a food you can't live without, write it down in the treat blank. However, do not land at your destination and beeline it for that treat. If you do that, you will be on a bender eating that "white" or sugary food for the remainder of your trip. Regret over not tasting a certain food will morph into regret from overdoing it. I say, save your treat card for the end of the trip, a day or two before you depart. You can play, it just needs to be delayed or else you risk the F-its.

BEWARE OF THE F-ITS

I have no problem cursing in real life but don't think I should here, and I'm not sure why. Let's pretend it's a few days into a vacation or work trip; you're eating a little too much here and there and feeling down on yourself. Never ever say, "When I get home I'll eat well" or "There's only a few more days" or any version of those. That's an F-it mindset. Nobody eats perfectly when they're away, but there is a tremendous difference between imperfection and overindulgence. F-its when you're a little off give you the license to eat more and worse. Remind yourself of your Anchor Behavior and focus there. Rein it in, whether it's dessert, the bread basket, or drinking, and keep that on track for the remainder of the trip. Or, as a client from Texas always says, "Get back on the diet horse."

If I had to pick one day that trips up travelers' eating, it would be the day you head home. Whether you've been eating well or with abandon, it's easy to get sucked into the last-hurrah Cinnabon. I had a running coach once scream "Finish strong" as I anxiously eyed the finish line at the end of a marathon. Let yourself smell the Cinnabon, but keep walking. Unlike the local flavors mentioned earlier, there is nothing treatworthy in the airport. It takes three hours and forty-five minutes, or almost a marathon, to burn off that end-of-trip-splurge Cinnabon, so finish strong.

Travel Glad Libs

If you travel more than a couple of times a year and need help with travel eating, try a little Mad Libs–like exercise I call Glad Libs before hitting the road. Filling in the blanks makes a potentially loosey-goosey trip feel orderly.

- I will do _____ Whole Foods Days before or after my trip to counteract vacation eating.
  (Insert "1" or "2.")

- My biggest food challenge when I go away is _____ , without a doubt.
  (Choose one: airport food, work meals, booze, mini-bar, sleep, or other.)

- I will hold myself to _____ boozy drinks per week, no matter how many my friends and colleagues have.
  (Insert "7" or less.)

- I'll commit to _____ minutes of exercise per week, regardless of hotel gym size or cleanliness.
  (Insert "100" or more.)

- I will _____ daily to keep me on a schedule.
  (Insert your Anchor Behavior.)

- I need flexibility when it comes to _____ _____.
  (Insert your Flex Area.)

- I will limit my travel treats to _____ per trip, even though I'll want more.
  (Insert a number equal to or less than the number of Whole Foods Days.)

Twelve

Pre-Beach Procedures, aka the Drastic Chapter

Dieting is the only game where you win when you lose.
—KARL LAGERFELD

One day I was in my office discussing weight goals with a new client. We talked about her "acceptable" weight, which she said was 125 pounds. She pinpointed 120 as her "amazing weight." "Of course, if I'm going to be in a bathing suit, I need to go a few pounds lower." "Of course," I replied, "everyone knows that."

Bathing suits seem to elicit some of the most extreme weight-related fear, but drastic measures are also appropri-

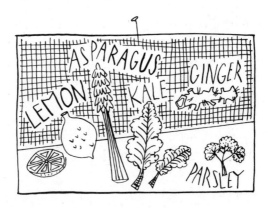

ate for weddings, reunions, or any occasion for which you feel you want to look your best and then some. In general, I pride myself on being practical; there is nothing gimmicky about my diet advice. However, there are times when sane or reasonable isn't going to get you where you want to go fast enough. Drastic measures are best used when you have a firm deadline. Pull out the stops seven days before your departure. Any longer and either drastic will shift into semidrastic or your results will dwindle. Drastic weeks are not the time to be overly social unless your friends want to come over and be drastic with you. I also suggest saving severe for a maximum of four times per year.

This question on the Foodtrainers blog captures the mind-set of a pre-beach person:

> My husband and I are heading to Hawaii for vacation. So I have a week before I leave for the beach. I've been pretty good about keeping to the food plan, but I'd love hints about what to do to maximize beach body potential. And I'm not looking for a miracle, I just want to up the ante. I don't want my mom to suggest that I look like a beached whale, which she has been known to do.

My reply:

Wow, Hawaii sounds fantastic but even more fantastic if you're feeling your best. And let's face it, whether it's your mom or your friends, other people do look at us, and though we deny it, we care what they think. With the trip a week away we don't have time for moderate. Drastic doesn't last, but there's a time for it and the time is now. So what does upping the diet ante look like? Here are the seven LBT pre-beach procedures:

1. **Eliminate.** Nope, I'm not talking about pooping (although it does improve the way you feel in a swimsuit; more on that later). I am talking about what you need to eliminate from your diet in the days before the beach. After all, what would a short-term plan be without some good old sacrifice and deprivation? You have your original No list (see page 12); now we're building on that list:

- *Skip sweet and wheat.* Sweet includes nutrition bars, dark chocolate, and treats normally allowed but not on the menu this week with the exception of fruit. You're already skipping gum and mints, right? (No list items.) Condiments are sneaky sweet sources, so no ketchup, hoisin, or barbecue sauce. Wheat refers to all wheat, sprouted or not.
- *Skip anything packaged* with more than two ingredients (eggs in a carton are okay; chips—and this means even healthy chips such as kale chips—are not).
- And while you're at it, *skip the 3 C's:* canned (or smoked) food, carbonated beverages, and all cocktails.
- *Nuts and cheese are also no-no's.* These are the two foods that can stall weight loss if portions are not exactly right. They are too risky right now.

Err on the side of skinny. If you have a question about whether something is okay to eat, assume it is not. I know eliminating doesn't always sound awesome, but this is completely temporary. As you shed the pounds, the eliminating will feel worthwhile.

2. **Blast the bloat.** In the short term you aren't focusing on losing huge amounts of body fat. Even if you are focused on it, it's not really possible in one week. However, there's

a big difference in feeling swollen versus sleek. My five favorite dietary de-bloaters (how is this word not in the dictionary?) are the following:

Asparagus

Dandelion greens

Parsley

Lemon

Ginger

These foods act in different ways to extinguish that extra layer—you know that layer. Potassium helps you shed sodium, or salt; parsley is a concentrated source of potassium though it's also in dandelion greens. Prebiotics in foods such as asparagus help feed the healthy gut bacteria, or probiotics. (Bad bacteria lead to bloat.) Have each of

Makes-You-Pee Tea

This homemade tea combines a few different de-bloating ingredients. If you don't have these on hand or want to "pee" with less preparation or effort, Yogi detox tea or Traditional Medicinals fennel tea can be substituted.

Minced parsley and stems (1 tablespoon per cup)
½ teaspoon fennel seeds
2 to 3 slivers peeled fresh ginger

Cover the parsley mixture in hot water, steep 5 to 10 minutes, and strain.

these every day in the week leading up to vacation. Yes, I said every day. Steam, grill, or roast two to three bunches of asparagus and eat them with your dinner every night. Add lemon slices to your water bottle. Parsley can be chopped into salads or boiled for a tea. And dandelion and avocado salad makes a great daily pre-beach lunch; both ingredients are found in the Drastic Salad (page 181).

Sorry if these aren't your favorite foods. While you may not find them the most delicious, de-bloating most certainly is.

3. **Disrobe.** It's very difficult (okay, traumatizing) to go from turtlenecks and boots to swimsuits and sunscreen. For all intents and purposes, we are all but naked on the beach unless you're like me, hidden securely beneath your cover-up du jour. The truth is there's little secrecy in a swimsuit. Your shape is your shape, and it will soon be out for everyone to see. What to do? We say practice! My brilliant intern Lisa mentioned, "I know this is pretty extreme, but in the days leading up to the beach, my roommate actually puts on her bathing suit when she gets home from work until she goes to bed. That is the time of day that she is most prone to overeating, and she knows she will make better choices if she's wearing the exact suit she wants to be in at the end of the week." I love this, and it works really well. It also helps you practice good posture, an easy slimming strategy if ever there was one. Sure, you can post a photo of a bathing suit on the fridge, but if you want to drive the message home, disrobing it is.

4. **Exit the elliptical.** Ever seen a friend you haven't seen in a while and they look great, amazing, lean, and just different? When you ask how they did it or what they changed, did they ever say they started to use the Precor? Or that they've been walking? I am not saying these forms

Juicy Snacks

In New York City, juice places are popping up everywhere; it's a trend I wholeheartedly support. One local juice chain mentioned they'd love a shop at every subway stop. While I'm thrilled to have something opening other than banks and coffee places, if juice-o-mania hasn't hit where you live, there's no reason why you can't juice yourself. When you see how much produce goes into one cup of juice, you'll understand how nutrition-packed it is.

You would have to eat nine cups of kale to get the calcium and iron in a 16-ounce green juice. If you're ready to point out to me that juice doesn't have the fiber of the whole vegetable, my answer is that that's exactly why you want to include it in your pre-beach plan. There's no digestive distress, but instead a healthy IV of goodness entering your body with no resistance or fiber to slow it down. You can pack juices with anti-inflammatory ingredients such as ginger, basil, parsley, lemon, and turmeric. Cilantro is another great herb; in particular, for frequent fish eaters, cilantro can bind mercury as it is digested. Enjoy your juices between meals because green juice, coconut water, and kombucha are your only snacks when you're going drastic. You'll find details on how to make Bikini Greenie (a drastic juice) on page 179.

Have at least one green juice daily in the week before your trip. If you don't own a juicer, you can blend ingredients and then strain off the juice. Or you can purchase a green juice. Make sure it only has one fruit added other than lime or lemon; you want a veggie-based juice, not a fruit juice. The only problem with purchasing your juice is that it won't taste as good as the Bikini Greenie.

of exercise are useless. You want to raise your good cholesterol? Ease your way into exercise? De-stress? That's one thing. You want to feel less lumpy in a swimsuit? Then you need more. *Run, spin, use the stair climber (looks like a staircase), jump rope, or do whatever form of exercise you hate or feel is "too hard." Do this six days a week (Aren't I nice? You get a day off!) for forty-five to sixty minutes.* Do it in your swimsuit for bonus points.

I also consulted one of my favorite yoga and barre instructors, Katrina Cydylo, for her opinion on the best yoga poses for bloat and "getting things going." She first suggested any variation of a twist. "The simplest and probably most relaxing is just lying on your back, arms out, and dropping your knees to one side. (It's more effective to twist the knees to the left side first so the ascending colon is being compressed.) Focus on taking deep breaths there for a minute or so, then switch sides. The other useful pose is just child's pose (kneel on a soft surface resting your rear end on your heels, exhale, and lower your forehead toward the ground with your arms outstretched over your head). Breathe there for a couple minutes; these work because you're massaging your intestines."

Do your most dreaded form of cardio, follow it with one of these chosen poses, and you've upped the exercise ante.

5. **Work that water.** Researchers can debate the amount of water we need to drink for optimal health, but in the meantime, I'll tell you how much H_2O you need to look

your best—a lot. I suggest 96 ounces daily of a combination of water with a cup or two of Teas' Tea green tea and homemade Makes-You-Pee Tea. It's counterintuitive, but water helps you lose water. And if we're dehydrated, sometimes we're tempted to eat when we actually need to drink, so just drink up in the first place.

6. **Include Super Power Foods.** When we're upping the ante, every ingredient counts. Regular, healthy foods are fine for regular days, but pre-beach you need Super Power Foods. You have your de-bloating tea (Makes-You-Pee Tea) and Bikini Greenie; here are a few other additions:

- *Virgin coconut oil:* The type of fat (lauric acid) in coconut oil is readily used for energy and less likely to be stored as fat. Studies have shown that virgin coconut oil decreases abdominal fat and produces greater weight loss than other oils. Do not toss the olive oil, but pre-beach use coconut oil for cooking eggs, add 1 teaspoon to smoothies, or melt over warm asparagus.
- *Apple cider vinegar:* Remember vinegar from the pantry list? One to two tablespoons of vinegar, such as Bragg's or Eden apple cider vinegar, decreases fat storage and increases weight loss. It's acetic acid, the main component of vinegar, that has this super power.
- *SoCal Cleanse organic protein and detox powder:* There are a lot of iffy products sold with *detox* as part of the name; this is not one of them. This organic hemp-based powder is rich in omega-3s. It also contains ingredients to assist digestion and improve liver function (the liver is our body's detoxifier).

7. **Close the kitchen at 6.** There is nothing gained from late-night eating, and the sooner the kitchen is closed, the better your weight loss will be.

**Kosher for Pre-Beach/Drastic Cheat Sheet and
Shopping List**
Stick to these foods and these foods only:

Fruits: lemon, limes, grapefruit, watermelon, papaya, avocado

CHECKLIST
ASPARAGUS, KALE
LEMONS AND GINGER

Vegetables: dandelion greens, microgreens, kale, fennel, fennel seeds, fresh
herbs (parsley, basil, cilantro, mint), asparagus, artichokes, radishes, cucumbers, celery, onions, garlic, ginger

Grain: quinoa (two servings per week but not in
the forty-eight hours be-
fore your trip; the only
grain—technically a seed—
permitted on the drastic plan; it
made the cut because of its potassium and magnesium content)

Beverages: Makes-You-Pee Tea, kombucha, green
juice, Harmless Harvest Coconut Water

Protein: SoCal Cleanse powder, fish, omega-3 eggs

Super Power Foods: coconut oil, apple cider vinegar, hot
sauce, cacao nibs

Dr. Seuss may not have been talking diets (though
Green Eggs are drastic-approved), but he knew what he
was saying:

You're off to Great Places!
Today is your day!
Your mountain [or swimsuit] is waiting,
So . . . get on your way!

A Sample Day in the Life of Drastic

The key to drastic is to stick to the Kosher for Pre-Beach/Drastic Cheat Sheet. I know how excuses work, and you do not need a blender, juicer, or coconut oil to feel self-confident in a swimsuit. Eliminate the 3 C's, up the exercise ante, and close the kitchen at 6, and great things will happen.

You can substitute as you wish, but keep to the ingredients on the Kosher for Pre-Beach/Drastic Cheat Sheet.

- Breakfast: 2 eggs and 5 asparagus spears, 1 teaspoon coconut oil with green tea or black coffee
- Midmorning: Bikini Greenie
- Lunch: Drastic Salad with 2 tablespoons avocado dressing
- Midafternoon: Kombucha or coconut water
- Dinner: 6 p.m. SoCal Shake (see page 180)
- Evening: Makes-You-Pee Tea

Thirteen

Holy Holiday Hazards

*People are so worried about what they eat
between Christmas and the New Year, but they
really should be worried about what they eat
between the New Year and Christmas.*

—ANONYMOUS

From one extreme to the other, swimsuits to Santa . . . In terms of Holiday Hazards, I'm going to go out on a limb and assume you know that sweet potato pie, matzo ball soup, and eggnog aren't slimming selections (see our Holiday Food Hall of Shame if you are suffering from treat amnesia). However, with the holidays, it's not just about the calories or the food. There's a reason why this chapter comes at the end of the book. Holidays are *The Little Book of Thin* final exam of sorts. There are family dynamics (pass the wine, please), traditional treats imbued with sentimental value, hours spent traveling, and lots of idle time once you're at your destination. Uh-oh, where's the nutrition panic button?

Holiday Problem Solving

Regardless of your religion or which holidays you celebrate, increasingly, most holidays are recognized by everyone. I will hear, "I'm not Jewish, but I saw matzo at the store; is it healthy?" It isn't, but it's around each and every spring. Holiday situations occur time and time again. You may not have realized it, but I would bet you'll find yourself nodding as you read on. Here are some common hazards and plans for conquering them.

PROBLEM: HOLIDAY BULGEOPHOBIA

Holidays have a ridiculously bad reputation when it comes to your weight. I find that some clients are worked into a tizzy before the holiday even "rolls" around. Catch yourself if you utter "I always gain weight this time of year" or "When I'm around my family I _____." I'm not saying you're wrong, but we have to recognize what can be somewhat Pavlovian food behavior. There's that defeatist diet-y thinking in all of us that can be very dangerous.

Solution: Where there's celebratory, there should also be spartan. Instead of bracing for indulgent impact, take precautionary eating measures. If holidays are synonymous with treats, you need to make room for them, literally. *Pick one to two days in the week before the holiday, mark them with an S in your calendar, and keep these days spartan.* Skip all grains and added sugar and work out for sixty minutes per day (as well as your Ten Steps to Svelte). If you implement a couple of these austerity days per week pre-holiday, you'll balance out the Christmas cookies and won't get mistaken for Santa.

Second, is there a time of day or scenario that's most tempting for you when it comes to the holidays? One client's family has a habit of heavy hors d'oeuvres in the afternoon during the holidays. Hors d'oeuvres do a lot of people in. There's cheese and salami, drinks and chips. This is more than enough to make a meal of, but then they sit down to dinner. We strategized that she'd limit herself by putting a few items on a cocktail napkin and skipping alcohol until she got to the dinner table. No cocktails at cocktail hour may sound illogical, but it's actually the opposite.

Another notoriously tricky time is during cleanup. While you're clearing plates or putting food away, your guard is down. It's easy to grab a few bites here, and things you may not have even had during the meal itself. Pinpoint where your celebration tends to take an unhealthy turn, and then you can troubleshoot.

PROBLEM: SLIM (HEALTHY) PICKIN'S

It's hard to believe in 2014 that someone can compose a menu with zero regard for health, but it happens, and it happens a lot for holiday meals. Even my mother uses my grandmother's stick-of-butter recipes and justifies it as "traditional" and therefore okay. For some reason, even people who in general eat fairly well choose to entertain in a more indulgent manner. Parents also make foods they feel are their children's favorite, which seems so kind, but if you're watching what you're eating, tell Mom she doesn't have to make the muffins or cookies you loved when you were eight.

Solution: Take sides. I remember meeting with a client right before Thanksgiving; I asked her what she planned to bring to the meal. "I am the cupcake girl," she reported. While I have no doubt her cupcakes are delicious, they certainly don't help her weight loss cause. I told her she should be the Brussels sprouts or green beans girl instead. Bringing a veggie side dish or crudité platter selfishly ensures a healthy component in the meal. You are not forcing your mindfulness on others. You're just making sure there's something you can eat. And if you are staying with relatives, offer to cook something for the house during your stay.

Holiday Treats

This is one of my favorite holiday emails:

> *What do I do about Thanksgiving? My happiest day involves giant bowls of mashed potatoes. I could eat my body weight in mashed potatoes given the opportunity. I don't really eat many other sides, just potatoes with a side of turkey. Do I splurge for the one day? I'm very stressed out about it.*

I'll offer up an example from my family. My sister makes trifle every year. It's beautiful and everyone loves it, but it's just not my thing. And each year when I say, "It looks amazing, but the gluten—I can't," she comes right back, honoring her role as the family food pusher, and tells me, "Sure you can" or "What difference will a little make?" Maybe she's channeling those bridesmaids.

On the other hand, eggnog is something I dream about. One person's eggnog is another's mashed potatoes. *Practice Treat Training*; preselect that holiday dish you must have, but heed the treat criteria.

To the reader: I don't know what you weigh, but a "body" of mashed potatoes will not leave you feeling happy (not to fantasy-bust). If it's "go mashed potatoes or go home," you can have a quarter of a plate of those buttery spuds: a portion. If there is an unadulterated vegetable side, eat as much of that as you do the potatoes, and have that turkey too.

What are the holiday foods you can't pass up? There are very few foods we each would say we'd have to consume "on our happiest day" or "for our last meal." Make it a mission to seek out the best version of those one or two foods and call it a day. Forgo whatever "trifle" is for you; it's not worth it. Reduce your portion size and savor your favorites, make the next meal on track, and the stress is gone.

PROBLEM: THE FOOD PUSHER

I tend to think every family has a food pusher, and for some reason mothers-in-law are commonly in this category. Food pushers have been known to ask, "Is that all you're eating?" or "How come you didn't try my potatoes?" Worst of all, they may plate food for you. Food pushers can be so pushy, it's important to expect to be pushed and know how you'll respond.

Solution: You can accept without needing to ingest. Whether it's a welcome cocktail or a piece of pie, radar is up for who accepts and who declines the food and drink. Politely receive your plate of food or glass of wine and, as I've mentioned, nobody will notice what you actually consume. A second, more aggressive route is to be honest and polite but push back: "It's so delicious, but I think I've had enough." It's always good to throw in a compliment while refusing food.

PROBLEM: HONESTY ISN'T ALWAYS THE BEST POLICY

You've been planning your holiday meal for months, but your mother says your turkey is dry or worse and starts passive-aggressively basting your oven contents. Or maybe your Aunt Ellen says you've "filled out," which we know is relative code for "porked up." It's July as I type this, but I find myself craving Christmas cookies just thinking about holiday dynamics. Familial criticism and conflict are responsible for boatloads of holiday calories.

Solution: Planning for disparagement defuses it. Once a critic, always a critic. We all have a mother who thinks she knows best, or an Aunt Ellen. Just as you pick out a holiday outfit or enter an address into your GPS, bolster yourself for the family fallout. Even if you cook a perfect meal or feel fantastically fit, do not expect the control freak or resident assessor to notice or change. If you are hosting the event and know that something someone does or says tends to upset the apple (or apple pie) cart, you can request a dietary no-fly zone of sorts. "Really looking forward to seeing you, but let's save diet talk for another day." Or simply brace yourself for the emotional impact.

I have a client with a tough-cookie mother. She and her sister have a running joke for family get-togethers. They've created this partner-in-criticism, strip-strategy game. Every time the mother makes a negative comment, one of them removes something (a watch or hair clip, for starters). It keeps it fun, and after years of playing this game, their mother still hasn't figured it out.

PROBLEM: UNBUTTONING YOUR PANTS IN INAPPROPRIATE PLACES WITH SERIOUS REGRET

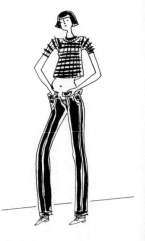

Holiday foods are rich, and for many of us holidays are the days we relax our food rules. However, there's a difference between bending the rules and busting loose. Though holidays each come once per year, there's a whole year of various holidays and special events. You can't indulge on all of them.

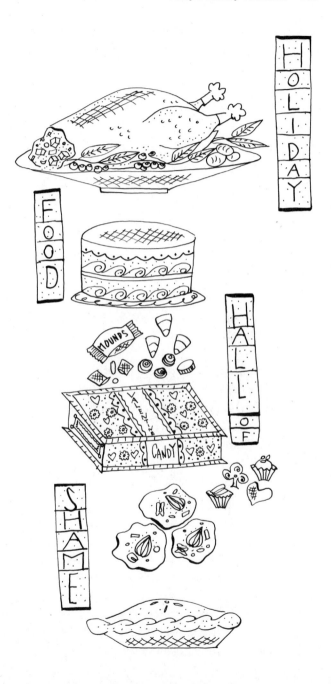

Holiday Food Hall of Shame

Here's the deal: We know Halloween candy isn't good for us. And while we can dissect calories and sugar and find the "better" selections, that doesn't mean they're green-lighted. At this point in the book, you know the LBT-approved foods. Having said that, every holiday I'm asked "What's the worst?" or "How bad is brisket?" So here you go. I'm not here to lay guilt (that's what relatives are for); if you see an item on this list you can skip, do so. If you see one of your favorites listed, know to watch yourself; the first taste is always the best.

ONE YEAR, TEN HOLIDAYS, TEN FOODS THAT *AREN'T* GOING TO MAKE YOU THIN

- **Valentine's Day:** Just because dark chocolate has health benefits doesn't mean the whole chocolate category gets a pass. That red heart-shaped box is synonymous with Valentine's Day . . . but there is nothing lovable about its nutrition info unless you're crushing on trans fats. You deserve better.
- **Passover:** If you've sat through a Seder, you know there's required drinking. Really, there's only required sipping; it doesn't have to be a week's worth of wine per night.
- **Easter:** Adults (and children, for that matter) don't need to eat Peeps with multiple sweeteners, pork-derived gelatin, preservatives, dyes, and 8 teaspoons of sugar for four bunnies. Don't even try the once-a-year rationale; there are now Peeps for other holidays too. If you steer clear of the *kids'* candy, there's

approved options such as ham, often asparagus, and let's not forget the Easter eggs.

- **Fourth of July:** Summer barbecues are relatively easy to make over in a healthy manner. Grill some chicken, eat some watermelon . . . what's so hard? Well, if there's fried chicken and you have a piece, one piece, it's over 400 calories and something I can suggest only if you crave intestinal fireworks.

- **Rosh Hashanah:** Carefully consider noodle kugel. A single serving has between 400 and 500 calories.

- **Yom Kippur:** I have a client who's a rabbi. When we discussed Yom Kippur one year, he told me he thought it made no sense to overdo it when you "break fast"; after all, you've spent the day atoning. If you wouldn't end a juice cleanse with a bagel, why load yourself up after a potentially religiously in-duced weight loss day? One bagel with cream cheese, lox, and a slice of tomato is almost 800 calo-ries. Remember, bagels are not for thin people, or even fasting people who want to be thin.

- **Halloween:** I'm not a fan of listing the best of the worst. Sure, 3 Musketeers and York Peppermint Patties have fewer calories than my two favorites, Almond Joy and Butterfinger, but with Halloween it's the tiny "fun size" or "mini" sizes that are the big-gest tricks. A few bite-size sweets add up to one full-size bar, and when would you ever eat that? As long as we're talking Halloween, there is a nutri-tional standout: Don't get lazy and toss those pump-kin seeds; save them and roast them. That's what you should munch on while you're waiting for the trick-or-treaters.

- **Thanksgiving:** The "standouts" here are stuffing (aptly named) and pecan pie. Just those two items add up to 800 calories for relatively small portions. If you love both of these, choose between loves; trust me, you'll be thankful. Sure, pumpkin pie is better, but a better pie? Turkey is the way to go, and go crazy; dark meat is the least of your worries at this meal.

- **Hanukkah:** Let's look at latke calories. Have I mentioned that potatoes are the food that's most correlated with weight gain? And when we fry them it only gets worse. One serving of latkes can have a miraculous 750 calories. I know oil has significance when it comes to Hanukkah, but there's no need to drown yourself in oil in order to celebrate that the oil burned for eight days. Let's light the menorah but bake the latkes.

- **Christmas:** With cream, alcohol, and sugar, one of my loves—eggnog—tops the Christmas (worst) list with over 400 calories per serving. You must make room for this type of calorie bomb. There's no mashed potatoes, dessert, or much of anything if you want to enjoy a little bit of eggnog. We can indulge, but we have to be mature about it.

Solution: Commit to the One Plate Rule. This is my number one holiday planning tip and a good rule for any buffet situation. Before taking your food, observe the offerings and formulate your strategy. Half your plate should be vegetables (ideally the green kind, perhaps the veggies you contributed as "green beans girl") or salad, even if you have to steal the garnish from something. One-quarter of your plate should be protein and another quarter can be grains. Eat your vegetables first; this aids digestion and fills you up on fiber. Savor this plate of holiday goodness because *there are no second helpings at dinner on this plan.* This rule works well in different food situations. The "hors d'oeuvres" client mentioned earlier used a cocktail napkin for her "one plate." It works no matter how challenging the food situation. The real celebration is that the One Plate Rule leaves you feeling light and self-righteous. Unbuttoning is over.

PROBLEM: GYMLESSNESS

Many of us are spoiled (my hand is raised). We have gyms or fitness studios we go to. Some of you may have additional fitness facilities at your workplace. When we travel, most hotels have gyms, even if some are creepy and unappealing. Then the holidays come and you're visiting your parents or in-laws in suburban Ohio or pretty much suburban anywhere and there's no gym, spin class, or trainer for miles. Or, if there is a gym, it's closed for the holidays when you need it most. There may be a stationary bicycle or NordicTrack; these lurk in many basements (if you're twentysomething you may have no idea what the heck a NordicTrack is) but may have been broken for years now, just sort of a souvenir from healthier times.

Solution: Don't be an exercise snob. Pack your sneakers, workout clothes, and iPod. Even if it's too cold or not as good a workout, commit to walking the day of the holiday *and* the day after. If you're thinking that walking isn't the best form of exercise, I agree with you. However, walking or other seemingly subpar exercise can clear your head, which is oh-so-important when surrounded by family or exploding from togetherness. Walking can also counter that diet-y black-or-white, on-or-off cycle that we're all guilty of. If you throw in some crunches and push-ups (there are fun push-up apps), you may burn off those cocktails.

PROBLEM: PROCRASTINEATING

ProcrastinEATING happens when you feel as if you had a large holiday meal and that you've blown it as far as your food plan goes. This is related to the on-or-off switch I mentioned with exercise. The procrastinEATER says, "On Monday I will be good" or "When I get home, I will get back on track" or, most dangerous of all, "Come January first, I'll start with a clean slate." ProcastinEATING is closely related to the F-its but can be more damaging because over the holidays you're surrounded by stuffing or latkes or pie.

Solution: Nip it in the bud. It's often not the holiday meals that do people in. It's the leftovers and the couple of days following the meal and the towel getting thrown in. If you are off track, regroup at the next meal and plan your food for the day following Rosh Hashanah, Thanksgiving, or Christmas. Whether it's Halloween candy or kugel, *keep holiday treats to the holidays themselves*. Depending on the holiday, tell yourself you can have a festive food on Christmas, but nothing the next day—December 26 isn't a holiday (at least, not in the United States). And watch the "pretzel logic"—that is, thinking you can't dispose of items because other family members may want them. Chances are your kids will forget about treats after twenty-four hours; we all know where treats retained "for the kids" end up.

Weddings and Funerals

Like holidays, weddings and funerals take us out of our day-to-day routines. You have to be at certain places at certain times; there's the family variable too, but weddings and funerals come with their own specific food challenges. For holidays, you have a general idea when the meal will be served. With weddings and funerals, the timeline is not your own and often unknown. Unlike a holiday meal, there's no ducking out to get something in another room or outside. You're pretty much held captive.

With weddings, a huge challenge can be budgeting alcohol over a long day or night. Throw in the extra fact that, at all but your cheapest functions, there's an open bar inviting you to overdo it. Then there's the issue of being seated at tables with people you may not know. Sure, family has its issues, but strangers? Sometimes your entrée can seem your only escape.

On the other end of the get-together spectrum, when someone dies, all anyone wants to do is bring you any and every food imaginable. Everyone is so concerned that the grieving will starve that they could practically kill them with calories. And when you're trying to support someone who has experienced a great loss, you often feel as though you don't know what to do or say. And so when you're offered a plate of food, it's easy to figure that's one way of acting correctly.

LBT WEDDING AND FUNERAL SOLUTIONS

- **The perfect clutch:** As one client said, the biggest wedding challenge is finding a bag that is formal enough, is cute enough, matches enough wedding-appropriate clothing, and yet can still fit a protein bar or other "sneak food" inside it when you're in for a long night.

- **Pre-think drinks:** I don't care how old you are; for some reason an open bar can be challenging. At many events there are waiters with trays of wine or champagne encouraging you to celebrate. Things can get Jerry Springer–like very quickly with the emotions of a big day and too much chardonnay. I suggest a two-drink limit for women and three for men, even if it's an all-day affair.
- **Dancing beats dessert:** The upside of the wedding is that there's built-in exercise. You don't have to be the dancey type (I'm not) but if it's that or sitting with the bride's father's accountant, Gangnam Style it is (or even the Macarena; seems nothing goes out of fashion when it comes to wedding music).
- **Best buffet tactic:** I can't say it enough: the One (reasonable) Plate Rule.
- **The funeral rule:** People want to comfort you or be comforted, but that doesn't mean you have to eat their potato salad even if the church ladies made it. No eating is mandatory.

The last thing on your mind with weddings and funerals is food, which is exactly why you need these LBT reminders.

Try Your Holiday Hotline or TIDEI

Whether it's a holiday, a wedding day, or just another day, if you're on Twitter, I'm here for you (and if not, so sorry). When you're tempted to get carried away, simply use the hashtag #TIDEI, which stands for *tweet it, don't eat it*. Tweet to @Foodtrainers and I'll tweet you off the food ledge.

By now, I hope you see that the thing about holidays or weight loss eating in general is that your success doesn't depend on doing everything right. If that were the case, nobody, no matter how metabolically gifted, would be thin. Getting to your "goal weight" or "getting leaner" or any measure of progress with food rests on making headway in the areas or scenarios that continually trip you up. We all have them and now you're on your way, armed with your *Little Book of Thin*, to solve them.

Fourteen

Thintastically Ever After

In the Middle Ages, they had guillotines,
stretch racks, whips and chains.
Nowadays, we have a much more effective
torture device called the bathroom scale.
—STEPHEN PHILLIPS

By now, you're in the planning groove with food shopping, cooking, snacking, and socializing. You wear the (smaller) pants when it comes to your weight. If there's still an ounce of residual fear, that's okay. Confidence with food is hard to come by, and a drop of concern over regaining weight often helps keep you from doing just that. It takes continual practice with your LBT habits. I saved a couple of crucial areas for last, for your Plan-It-to-Lose-It commencement address.

Victory List

Most of us thrive on praise. I'm not talking empty compliments or Pollyanna-isms but honest, well-deserved positive feedback. Whether you're twenty-five or sixty-five, male or female, the gold star, pat on the back, or thumbs-up feels good . . . even if you have to give it to yourself. At the beginning of this book, I mentioned we all eat well until life gets in the way. Well, we can also get in our own way. Positivity needs to be part of your thin plan.

In our offices we have stickers. We have a "gold star"—actually a golden orange (from our logo; you can't forget branding). We have a golden frying pan for cooking progress, a golden suitcase for healthy travel, a golden wineglass for drinking within budget. Even clients who roll their eyes when I reward them end up asking if they get a sticker on future visits. But you don't need stickers to do this.

On your Menu Map or in your phone, keep a Victory List. Each day, think about what you did well. Maybe it's "skipped the bread basket" or "had one liter of water by lunch." If you're going to the effort to plan and organize, the scale is not the only judge (and we'll get to that in a minute). You know when you're improving, and when you take notice of this and remind yourself, you're going to do it more. When you're stuck on a diet indiscretion, unstick yourself by saying, "What am I doing well?" My clients come in wanting to confess their food sins, but we turn things around when I ask them to toot their own horn.

Weight Loss Commentary from "Friends"

As you work at implementing positivity, don't expect others around you to be rosy. When you're losing weight, there's another important nonfood variable to keep in mind and that's the unsolicited comments that "friends," coworkers, and family members make about your progress. Some people seek feedback from others. Early on, clients will say, "Nobody is noticing yet." However, it's a double-edged sword once they do notice. If nobody notices, then it's easy to infer that you aren't doing a good job and feel dejected. However, once the folks do realize that you're slimming down, watch out.

First, it's easy to loosen up once you're feeling physically better and others are telling you that you look good. I cannot say this strongly enough, but *if we cease to Foodtrain once we feel a bit better, we will return to feeling poorly.* And then there are the ridiculous things jealous or foolish people say when someone around them is losing weight (and they're not).

"You're disappearing," a colleague said to a determined client of mine who hasn't had an easy time in life. Her weight loss was just part of her journey, in which she was learning to take care of herself and go for things she really wanted. Her coworker had no way of knowing any of this, but I couldn't have scripted it better; she replied, "No actually, I'm appearing."

Oh my goodness, I've heard such silly things said to weight loss clients like, "Don't lose any more weight" or "You better be careful not to get too thin or you will start to look old." The list goes on. File this away as you proceed on your own journey. Your response to comments doesn't have to be eloquent; you actually don't even need to say anything at all. Just have confidence in the process and in yourself. It's always interesting to see who's really in your corner . . . as the corner starts to shrink.

Scale It Down

Perhaps you've been wondering how you know you're making progress. "Is this working?" "Am I doing this right?" Not to sound too Glenda the Good Witch, but I could argue that you already know how you're doing. When you stick to one Smart Snack in the afternoon, hit your cardio budget, and eat according to plan, whether you're socializing or traveling, you're "on" and it feels great. But then there's the dreaded scale question—should you weigh yourself?

I hate hedging, but it depends . . . For some of you reading this, the scale is your frenemy. While it appears to be useful, it may drive you crazy or determine whether you'll be in a good or bad mood, and for these reasons you may already have tossed it. Others of you may feel the scale keeps you sane and doesn't let you veer too far.

The scale can play games with your head much like the weight loss commentary I described earlier. There's a great *Cathy* cartoon about the scale. I don't recall the exact wording, but the strip showed Cathy getting on the scale, and the caption said something like "I lost weight, hooray, now I can eat something." The following panels had Cathy once again getting on the scale. Only this time, the caption indicated Cathy had gained weight. Her response was, "Oh well, this isn't working. I may as well eat something I shouldn't." Sound familiar? If the scale has this effect on you and can change your behavior for the day, it's not your friend, and I would suggest weighing yourself infrequently, once a month maximum.

I have even been known to stage scale interventions with clients. When half a session is monopolized by "I was 136.2 on Monday, but today I'm 137," it's energy that's diverted from strategizing and losing weight. I will request that the clients bring their scale to the next appointment. I don't give a reason for this. Funny enough, most "scale" people assume they are bringing their scale to be sure our scales match. I couldn't care less about that. When they show up, scales rolled in towels and stuffed into a shopping bag, I point to the corner of the office and tell them, "You can leave it there." They ask: "You're taking it?" I assure them that it's just for a week. The truth is, if you are a slave to the scale, you'll be more productive when it's gone. I have more than a few unclaimed and really nice devices hanging around because clients didn't want them back. They were empowered without them.

If this scale scenario resonated with you, you'll probably do better working on the Victory List or selecting a piece of reference clothing. Sure, many people have "skinny jeans," but your reference clothing can be a pair of fitted pants or a body-conscious dress. Men often use tuxedos for their reference clothing. If you can, pick something you remember feeling great in. Periodically try it on and see where you are. One client, a supersmart lawyer, came in one day and said, *I can get into my reference jeans but they are not ready for public consumption yet.* That's progress.

However, if you're someone who likes data and tracking weight, the scale may very well help you spot a trend before it gets out of hand. I'm not being sexist (or maybe I am), but men love numbers when it comes to weight. Whether it's the scale, body fat percentages, pedometers, you name it, I think the objectivity appeals to them. I had one client, a distance runner, who presented me with graphs of his daily weight over a ten-year period. If you're a passionate tracker, a daily weight is fine. It's fine to get on once a day, first thing before breakfast, sans clothes. Jumping on through-out the day is *not* okay—it's really a waste of time. I'd also advise against getting on the scale if you were on an air-plane or know full well you overindulged the day before. Give yourself twenty-four hours of normal eating and then weigh yourself.

Chances are this isn't your first diet "rodeo"; know your-self and choose one way to monitor progress. You decide if a daily weight, monthly weight, or reference clothing make the most sense for you.

The Maintenance Myth

As you use your Plan-It-to-Lose-It strategies and reap the weight rewards, you may be thinking, how does maintenance work? And that's just it: To maintain your weight takes work, but it's reasonable work. You don't resent (or maybe you do, but we still take it as a given) that you have to exercise in order to stay fit. The same thing goes for staying thin. There is no finish line where you are left to com-

---

Is My Scale Broken?

Avoid the "my scale may be broken" excuse and invest in a good scale if you plan on relying on it. All too often what we think we weigh is 5 to 10 pounds less than reality. For home use, a digital scale is best. *Consumer Reports* has shown that analog scales—you know, the old-school type with the dial—are often inaccurate. Eat Smart brand scales get top reviews in various rankings. Withings and Fitbit make Wi-Fi floor scales if you prefer something high-tech. Certain models will even email you based on your weigh-in. Some people love the feedback and encouragement this technology offers. I would stick with body weight because the body fat testing on home scales is easily skewed by hydration status, and readings can be imprecise and all over the place.

---

pletely wing it when it comes to your food choices. We know that story, and it results in feeling how you did when you bought this book (and others). Whether it's the Walk-through, one carb a day max, or dunch, you now have the tactics to handle any diet dilemma. That should feel good whether you have 20 or 0 pounds to lose. You have the strategy and information to weigh whatever you want to weigh. With *The Little Book of Thin* you can live thin-tastically ever after.

The (now smaller) End.

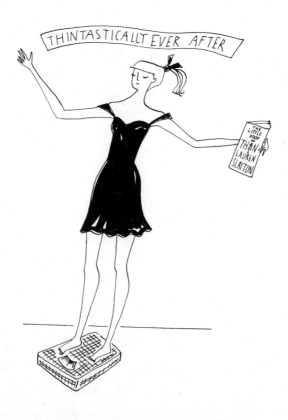

Three Ingredients, Three Ways

Rather than presenting all sorts of random recipes, I thought it best to pick a few key ingredients and show how they can be used in different ways. For example, if you cook a batch of quinoa, it can be used for the Spinach-Quinoa Cakes or the insanely tasty Miso Broccoli and Quinoa Salad. Following the basics and variations for quinoa, kale, and grilled chicken, you'll find recipes that solve each diet dilemma, many of which were mentioned in the text.

STARTER QUINOA

This method makes for fluffy quinoa; giving the quinoa a rinse before cooking improves the taste.

Makes 3½ cups or approximately 4 "fists"

2 cups water

1 cup quinoa, rinsed

¼ teaspoon Himalayan or Celtic sea salt

In a small saucepan, bring the water to a boil. Add the quinoa and salt. Reduce the heat to a simmer, cover, and cook until all the water is absorbed, about 15 minutes.

SPINACH-QUINOA CAKES

These protein-packed patties are perfect for lunch or even breakfast. To reheat, zap them in the microwave in 30-second intervals. When cooking, don't crowd the cakes in the pan. If necessary, sauté them in two batches.

Makes 4 servings

1½ cups cooked quinoa

1 egg white, beaten

1 tablespoon finely chopped jalapeño pepper (or to taste)

2 teaspoons Dijon mustard

10-ounce package frozen spinach, defrosted and well drained

½ teaspoon salt

1 teaspoon red wine vinegar

Freshly ground black pepper to taste

1 tablespoon extra virgin olive oil

In a large bowl, mix all of the ingredients except the olive oil together with a fork. Using your hands, form the quinoa mixture into 8 patties, about 2 inches across and ½ inch high.

Heat the olive oil in a large sauté pan (preferably nonstick) over medium heat. Sauté the patties until golden brown, 3 to 4 minutes on each side.

MISO BROCCOLI AND QUINOA SALAD

This salad will make you look forward to lunchtime all morning.

Makes 4 servings

3 tablespoons extra virgin olive oil

1 tablespoon white miso

2 tablespoons rice vinegar

2 cups cooked quinoa

3 cups steamed broccoli florets, roughly chopped

2 cups baby arugula

¼ cup raw sunflower seeds

¼ teaspoon salt

To make the dressing: In a small bowl, whisk together the olive oil, miso, and rice vinegar. Set aside.

In a large bowl, combine the quinoa, broccoli, arugula, and sunflower seeds. Add the dressing and the salt. Toss gently until combined.

STARTER KALE

Look for Lacinato kale, aka Tuscan kale, dinosaur kale, or cavalo nero. It is more tender and less bitter than its curly-leafed cousin. Substitute chicken broth or vegetable broth for the water to add extra flavor to this dish.

Makes 1 cup

1 tablespoon extra virgin olive oil

1 clove garlic, sliced

⅛ teaspoon crushed red pepper flakes (or to taste)

Kosher salt

1 bunch Lacinato kale, stems discarded and leaves roughly chopped (about 8 cups)

½ cup water (or broth, see above)

Freshly ground black pepper to taste

Heat the olive oil in a large sauté pan or Dutch oven. Add the garlic, red pepper flakes, and a pinch of salt. Reduce the heat to medium-low and cook gently for 5 minutes.

Add the kale to the pan. Cook for 5 minutes, stirring frequently.

Add the water, cover, and cook for 15 minutes. Season with ¼ teaspoon salt and black pepper to taste.

GREEN EGGS

My clients love these muffin-tin frittatas, and I love a high-protein "green" breakfast. These are as easy as 1-2-3 when you have the kale on hand.

Makes 4 servings

1 cup sautéed kale
4 eggs
¼ teaspoon salt
½ teaspoon smoked paprika
¼ teaspoon chili powder
Freshly ground black pepper to taste

Preheat the oven to 350°F. Spray four cups in a standard-sized muffin pan with organic cooking spray. Divide the kale between the muffin cups.

In a small bowl, whisk together the eggs, salt, paprika, chili powder, and black pepper to taste. Pour the eggs evenly over the kale in the muffin cups. Bake until just set, 15 to 20 minutes. Let the frittatas cool in the pan for 5 minutes, then gently remove.

KALE SLAW

Because this salad is composed of hearty vegetables, it will keep in the refrigerator for a couple of days.

Makes 6 servings

2 tablespoons extra virgin olive oil
2 tablespoons freshly squeezed lime juice
1 teaspoon Tabasco sauce (or to taste)
½ teaspoon salt
1 bunch Lacinato kale, stems removed and leaves thinly sliced (6 to 8 cups)
3 cups thinly sliced green cabbage, preferably Napa
2 carrots, shredded with a serrated peeler or sliced into thin strips
1 apple, cored and thinly sliced
⅔ cup roughly chopped fresh cilantro

In a small bowl, whisk together the olive oil, lime juice, Tabasco, and ¼ teaspoon of the salt.

In a large bowl, gently toss together the kale, cabbage, carrots, apple, and cilantro. Top with the dressing and the remaining ¼ teaspoon salt. Toss again.

STARTER CHICKEN CUTLETS

If you don't have a grill pan or an outdoor grill, simply sauté these cutlets on the stovetop. The chicken can be marinated for as briefly as 5 minutes to as long as 4 hours. If you're marinating the chicken for longer than 30 minutes, cover the bowl with plastic wrap and place it in the refrigerator.

Makes 4 cutlets

1 tablespoon extra virgin olive oil
Juice of 1 lemon
⅛ teaspoon crushed red pepper flakes
Salt
Freshly ground black pepper to taste
1 pound organic chicken cutlets

In a medium bowl, whisk together the olive oil, lemon juice, red pepper flakes, ¼ teaspoon salt, and black pepper to taste. Add the chicken cutlets and mix to make sure they are evenly coated with the lemon mixture. Let the cutlets marinate for up to 4 hours.

Heat a stovetop grill pan over medium-high heat. Remove the chicken from the marinade. Sprinkle both sides of each cutlet with salt and pepper to taste. Grill until cooked through, 3 to 4 minutes per side.

SOUPER EASY CHICKEN SOUP

Once your chicken is grilled, this soup comes together in 20 minutes. Add a dash of hot sauce for an
extra kick.

Makes approximately 3 servings

1 tablespoon extra virgin olive oil
½ medium yellow onion, chopped
2 carrots, chopped
2 stalks celery, chopped
3 cups low-sodium chicken broth
2 grilled chicken cutlets, shredded or diced
¼ teaspoon salt
1 tablespoon freshly squeezed lemon juice
2 cups baby spinach
Freshly ground black pepper to taste

Heat the olive oil in a medium pot. Add the onion, carrots, and celery. Reduce the heat to medium-low and cook
gently until the vegetables are tender, about 12 minutes.

Add the broth and bring to a boil. Add the chicken and
simmer for 5 minutes. Add the salt and lemon juice and
stir to combine. Add the spinach and black pepper to taste.

"GREEK" CURRIED CHICKEN SALAD

Serve this salad on baby spinach or arugula for more nutritional bang for your buck. The salad will keep in the fridge for 48 hours.

Makes 2 servings

¼ cup 2% plain Greek yogurt

1½ teaspoons Dijon mustard

1 tablespoon white wine vinegar

½ teaspoon curry powder

¼ teaspoon turmeric

¼ teaspoon salt

Freshly ground black pepper to taste

2 grilled chicken cutlets, shredded or diced

1 stalk celery, chopped

1 carrot, grated or chopped

½ apple, cored and chopped

1 scallion, chopped

In a small bowl, whisk together the yogurt, mustard, vinegar, curry powder, turmeric, salt, and black pepper to taste.

Place the chicken, celery, carrot, apple, and scallion in a medium-sized bowl. Add the dressing and toss. Taste for seasoning, adding salt and pepper if necessary.

HOW TO BOIL THE PERFECT EGG

When I first started my nutrition practice, I made the mistake of assuming that everyone knew how to boil eggs or steam vegetables. I soon learned that you cannot assume cooking skills, no matter how basic. And sometimes, even when we feel we know what to do, there are tricks or tweaks to improve on our method. Hard-boiling is botchable.

6 omega-3 eggs (chickens are fed flax, giving the eggs omega-3s)

Put the eggs into a pot just large enough to hold the eggs in a single layer with no stacking. Add enough water to just cover the eggs. Do not salt the water, as this can toughen the eggs. If your eggs float to the top of the water, they're too old to use.

Place the pot over medium-high heat.

The second the water starts to boil, remove the pot from the heat, cover the pot, and let the eggs sit. While it's definitely not the rumored 3 minutes, if you take a shower and dry your hair and come back to your eggs, they will be gray. My vote is for 12 minutes for medium eggs. Add 2 minutes if the eggs are extra large.

When the eggs are done resting, drain the water but keep the eggs in the pot. Run them under cold water for 2 minutes.

Here is the key to peeling eggs: Drain off any cold water, place the lid back on the pot, and shake the eggs in the pot for 30 seconds. The eggs will start to peel.

Finish peeling the eggs under cold running water. You can store hard-boiled eggs in a sealed container for up to a week.

Please Don't Say Steamed Vegetables Are Boring

There's a misconception that steamed vegetables are banal and tasteless, but this stems from the fact that not everyone knows how to make them properly. So if you're ending up with off-putting mush, you may be oversteaming or under-seasoning. Don't jump ship; steamed vegetables retain nutrients more than those cooked by many other cooking methods, and they're very versatile.

With so many foods available that are processed or overly (read: artificially) flavored, sometimes basic, unadulterated ingredients are best. It's sort of the food equivalent of the white button-down shirt.

Feel free to experiment, adding herbs such as thyme or rosemary to the water or throwing in a chunk of peeled ginger, pickle juice, wine, citrus, or citrus zest, though not necessarily all at once.

Here are the basics to help you get more veggies into your diet:

THE STEAMER

I steam my vegetables in an All-Clad steamer basket with a perforated bottom. You can also use a bamboo steamer, where vegetables are stacked; it's sort of the cooking equivalent of apartment living. Another option is the collapsible metal basket. The key here is to make sure the vegetables are above the water level.

THE LIQUID

Fill the pot with 1 to 2 inches of filtered tap water. You don't want all the water to evaporate while steaming or you'll burn your pot. Let the water come to a boil over medium-high heat before adding the vegetables.

THE VEGETABLES

Fill the steamer basket with vegetables; you can stack them even in a single basket, but don't overpack.

Different vegetables require different steaming times. If steaming more than one vegetable, add those that take longer, such as carrots or artichokes, first, and add those that cook quickly later.

Vegetables are cooked when they are fork-tender.

Sprinkle vegetables with Himalayan salt and, if you're eating them right away, toss with coconut oil or a sliver of pastured butter.

Store extra steamed vegetables undressed and use them in omelets, grain dishes, salads, or soups.

You'll soon learn how much cooking time it takes to make each vegetable fork-tender, but use the following chart as a guideline:

VEGETABLE	COOKING TIME
Artichokes	30 to 35 minutes
Carrots	12 minutes
Broccoli	5 to 7 minutes
Cauliflower	6 to 8 minutes
Kale	5 to 7 minutes
String beans	Less than 5 minutes
Spinach (and softer greens)	3 minutes

LBT STARTER SMOOTHIE

I've heard all sorts of complaints about smoothies from my clients. Some say they like to chew—something. Others claim they don't have enough time in the morning. To the chewers, I will remind you that we all like to chew. So use enough ice or frozen fruit to make the smoothie chewably thick—to the point you have to eat it with a spoon. To the time-strapped, have ingredients prepped or even put everything except the liquid in the blender the night before and leave it in the fridge. Smoothies are a delicious way to get protein, fluid, fruits, and vegetables in one glass. And they're great for weight loss.

For the protein powder I recommend Sunwarrior (hemp and pea protein), Tera's Whey (whey must be from grass-fed cows), or hemp protein powder. (Skip soy powders and whey protein that is not organic.)

Makes 1 smoothie

4 to 6 ounces unsweetened almond milk or water
1 scoop protein powder
1 cup fruit, fresh or frozen, cut up into chunks
1 handful greens (baby spinach and kale work well)
NuStevia (optional)

Place the ingredients in a high-powered blender (I find the Vitamix essential for making smoothies that contain greens) in the order given. Blend well and serve.

MATCHA COLADA

This smoothie is great for breakfast and is the ideal postworkout beverage. Matcha is a powdered green tea with even more antioxidants than a brewed cup of green tea. I love an organic brand called Do Matcha. Pineapple contains bromelain, an excellent remedy for swelling or inflammation, while papaya has an enzyme called papain, also used for sports injuries. Both coconut water and avocado provide potassium; avocado has some good fat to help absorb fat-soluble nutrients.

When you're thinking "I deserve a treat," here it is.

Makes 1 serving

4 to 6 ounces coconut water (or water)
½ teaspoon matcha powder
1 cup fresh or frozen pineapple or papaya
1 scoop protein powder (Sunwarrior or Tera's Whey)
1 cup greens (microgreens, spinach, or kale)
⅓ avocado, peeled and roughly chopped
1 slice peeled fresh ginger (the size of a penny)
1 handful ice cubes
6 drops NuStevia

Place coconut water (or water) in a high-powered blender followed by the other ingredients in the order given. Blend well and serve.

BIKINI GREENIE

This is the juice you want to make if there's a swim-suit in your future. It's also a delicious snack for less drastic days.

Makes 1 serving

3 cups kale, roughly chopped

2 cups watermelon, cubed

2 to 3 leaves fresh basil

1 lime with most of the peel sliced off

1 cucumber, cut in half

2 stalks celery

Fresh ginger, juiced microgreens, or dash of hot sauce afterward (optional)

Prepare and rinse all of the ingredients. Load all of the ingredients into a juicer (with the exception of hot sauce, if you are using it). Once juiced, give the liquid a stir and enjoy.

6 P.M. SOCAL SHAKE

On the drastic plan, this is dinner. No kidding.

When it comes to choosing almond milk for this, or any recipe, I'm being picky, but it's for your benefit. Read almond milk ingredients and choose one without carrageenan (such as 365 Whole Foods almond milk). Without getting too technical, carrageenan is used as a thickener but it's difficult to digest. No, thank you.

1 handful ice cubes

1–2 tablespoons SoCal Cleanse powder (or other hemp-based powder)

Fresh mint or mint extract

1 handful kale or spinach

Coconut oil

2 teaspoons cacao nibs

Unsweetened almond milk

NuStevia (optional)

Place the ingredients in a high-powered blender in the order given. Blend well and serve.

THIN-I-GETTE DRESSING

Thin-I-Gette beats bottled vinaigrette by a mile. There's no added sugar. Miso and vinegar are both "thinning" ingredients.

Makes about ¼ cup

1 tablespoon miso
2 tablespoons rice vinegar
¼ cup olive oil

Combine all ingredients in a small jar with a lid. Cover and shake.

DRASTIC SALAD WITH AVOCADO DRESSING

For me, this recipe epitomizes LBT eating. The Drastic Salad is as strict as you get "pre-beach," and yet you will never feel deprived eating it. This colorful salad is beautiful arranged on a plate or packed in layers in a jar for easy transport. Feel free to swap in lemon juice for the lime.

Makes 2 servings

For the dressing:

1 very ripe avocado
2 tablespoons freshly squeezed lime juice
2 tablespoons extra virgin olive oil
¼ teaspoon salt

For the salad:

2 cups dandelion greens, watercress, or baby arugula

½ cup roughly chopped Italian parsley

4 radishes, thinly sliced

4-inch piece of cucumber, preferably hothouse, thinly
    sliced

10 stalks steamed asparagus, chopped into 1-inch pieces

1 cup finely chopped fennel

To make the dressing: Mash the avocado in a small bowl. Using a fork or a whisk, mix in the lime juice, olive oil, and salt.

To make the salad: Divide the greens and parsley between two serving plates or containers. Top the greens with the radishes, cucumber, asparagus, and fennel, divided evenly between the two salads. Serve with the dressing.

PESTO TURKEY BURGERS

These are fantastic for lunch or dinner, or try making them in a smaller "slider" size for snacks. This is a recipe you'll want to double; it's a family favorite for us.

Makes 3 or 4 patties

1 pound organic ground turkey or chicken

2 tablespoons basil pesto

1 tablespoon shredded Parmesan

1 clove garlic, minced

1 pinch salt

Freshly ground black pepper to taste

In a large bowl, combine all of the ingredients. Form into 3 or 4 patties. Grill on a hot grill or grill pan for 10 to 13 minutes, turning once. Serve over arugula or on sprouted bread.

WEEKDAY TENDERLOIN

Preparing this pork tenderloin couldn't be easier, and the results are tender and flavorful. Put it in the oven, change your clothes, steam some vegetables, and dinner is served.

Makes 4 servings

2 tablespoons Dijon mustard
1 tablespoon extra virgin olive oil
2 tablespoons chopped fresh sage
1 pound organic pork tenderloin

Preheat the oven to 400°F. Line a baking sheet with parchment paper.

In a medium bowl, stir together the mustard, olive oil, and sage. Coat the pork tenderloin with the mustard mixture and place the pork on the baking sheet.

Roast until the temperature on an instant-read thermometer reaches 150°F when inserted into the thickest part of the tenderloin, 25 to 35 minutes, depending on the thickness of the pork.

Place the pork on a cutting board and cover loosely with foil. Let it rest for 10 minutes, carve, and serve.

SUPER BOWL STEW

French lentils are small green lentils that keep their shape when cooked. They are sometimes called lentils du Puy. Leftover stew can be refrigerated for three days or frozen for up to three months.

Makes 4 servings

2 tablespoons extra virgin olive oil

1 yellow onion, chopped

2 carrots, peeled and chopped

2 stalks celery, chopped

2 cloves garlic, minced

6 cups chicken or vegetable stock

¼ cup crushed tomatoes or 1 plum tomato, chopped

1½ cups green lentils, rinsed

1 tablespoon chopped fresh oregano

1 teaspoon salt

1 teaspoon balsamic vinegar

4 cups loosely packed baby spinach

Freshly ground black pepper to taste

In a large pot, heat the olive oil over medium-high heat. Add the onion, carrots, and celery. Reduce the heat to medium-low and cook gently until the vegetables are soft, but not brown, about 10 minutes. Stir occasionally to prevent burning. Add the garlic and cook for 2 more minutes.

Add the stock, tomatoes, lentils, oregano, salt, and vinegar. Increase the heat to high and bring the stew to a boil. Reduce the heat to a simmer and cover, cooking until the lentils are tender, about 55 minutes. Remove from the heat.

Add the baby spinach, stirring until it wilts. Season with black pepper to taste. Taste for seasoning, adding salt and pepper if necessary.

BEEF AND SPINACH "GREEN" BALLS

These meatballs get brightness from the lemon, tenderness from the mushrooms, and pep from the cayenne pepper, not to mention lots of vitamins and minerals from the spinach. Freeze leftovers by wrapping them individually in foil and then storing in a zip-top bag.

Makes 8 meatballs

1 tablespoon extra virgin olive oil

8 ounces cremini or button mushrooms, very finely chopped

¾ teaspoon kosher salt

1 pound organic grass-fed beef

1 egg, beaten

10 ounces frozen chopped spinach, thawed and excess liquid squeezed out

1 teaspoon lemon zest

¼ teaspoon cayenne pepper (optional)

Freshly ground black pepper to taste

Preheat the oven to 375°F. Line a baking sheet with parchment paper.

Heat the olive oil in a medium sauté pan over medium-high heat. Add the mushrooms and ¼ teaspoon of the salt and sauté until browned, about 7 minutes. Transfer to a medium bowl and allow to cool slightly.

Place the beef, egg, spinach, lemon zest, the remaining ½ teaspoon salt, cayenne pepper (if using), and black pepper to taste in a large bowl. Add the cooked mushrooms. Gently combine with your hands, taking care not to overmix. Divide the mixture into 8 meatballs and place them on the baking sheet.

Bake for 30 to 35 minutes, or until the meatballs reach 160°F on an instant-read thermometer.

ESSENTIAL POACHED SALMON

Prepare the salmon and sauce up to 48 hours in advance. This is the perfect "dunch" meal and a dish that tastes best cold or chilled. As long as your pot is big enough, you can poach additional salmon fillets at the same time. Just make sure they're in a single layer and that the liquid covers the fillets completely. The dill sauce is optional.

Makes 2 servings

For the salmon:

 1 bottle white wine
 2 quarts water
 ½ lemon, thinly sliced
 10 peppercorns
 2 (6-ounce) salmon fillets (preferably wild-caught), rinsed
 Kosher salt and freshly ground black pepper to taste

For the sauce:

 3 tablespoons 2% Greek yogurt
 ¼ cup finely chopped dill
 2 teaspoons white wine vinegar
 1 teaspoon Dijon mustard
 ¼ teaspoon kosher salt

To poach the salmon: In a large, wide pot, bring the wine and water to a simmer. Add the lemon slices, peppercorns, and salmon, skin side down. Keep the heat at a gentle simmer; bubbles should barely break the surface of the water. Cover and cook for 10 minutes. Remove the pot from the heat, remove the cover, and let the fish rest in the water for another 10 minutes. Transfer the fish to a plate. When it is cool enough to handle, remove the skin and sprinkle the salmon with salt and black pepper to taste. Refrigerate until chilled, at least 4 hours.

To make the dill sauce: Stir together the ingredients for the dill sauce. Taste for seasoning, adding more salt if necessary.

DATE-NIGHT SALMON

Impress your date with this one-dish dinner. To make the parchment packet, channel your elementary school self and cut out a giant heart. Or, if it's a first date, a rectangle is fine too.

Makes 2 servings

2 bunches baby bok choy, ends chopped off and split
    horizontally
2 (4- to 6-ounce) wild salmon fillets, skin removed
Salt and freshly ground black pepper to taste
1-inch piece ginger, peeled and cut into matchsticks
½ red bell pepper, cut into thin strips
2 scallions, chopped into ½-inch pieces
2 teaspoons rice vinegar

Preheat the oven to 450°F. Cut two pieces of parchment paper, about 18 inches long by 14 inches wide. Fold each piece of parchment in half and, using scissors, cut a large heart out of the paper. Place the hearts on a baking sheet and unfold them.

Lay one bunch of bok choy on each piece of parchment paper, close to the fold, as a "bed" for the salmon.

Top the bok choy with a piece of salmon and sprinkle the fish with salt and black pepper to taste.

Lay half of the ginger, half of the bell pepper, and half of the scallions on each salmon fillet.

Drizzle 1 teaspoon of rice vinegar over each fillet. To seal the packet, think fold and crease. Beginning at the top of the heart, fold and crease your way down, making sure the packet is completely covered. Twist the bottom of the heart to complete the seal. Repeat the process with the second piece of parchment and the remaining ingredients.

Bake the packets for 15 minutes. Let sit for 5 minutes before serving. Place the packets on plates and cut them open at the table for a dramatic, "steamy" presentation.

NO-FUSS FISH

If you are under the impression you can't cook fish at home, I'm here to prove you wrong. No-Fuss Fish is easy to prepare and clean up, and so light and un-fishy that you can eat it the next day. Feel free to double this recipe to feed a hungry family.

Makes 2 servings

2 tablespoons freshly squeezed lime juice

2 teaspoons extra virgin olive oil

2 (4- to 6-ounce) sole fillets

Salt and freshly ground black pepper to taste

2 tablespoons roughly chopped fresh cilantro

Preheat the oven to 400°F. Line a baking sheet with parchment paper.

In a small bowl, whisk together the lime juice and olive oil.

Place the fish on the parchment paper and season both sides with salt and black pepper to taste.

Bake the fish for 5 minutes. Pour the lime and olive oil mixture over the fillets and bake for 5 more minutes, or until the fish is just cooked through. Top with the cilantro.

Note: If you don't see sole at the market, you can substitute flounder, red snapper, or cod. The latter two might require a couple more minutes of cooking time.

SPICY SWEET POTATO FRIES

These sweet and spicy fries are crowd-pleasers. Serve on their own as a snack or as a "treaty" side dish.

Makes 3 servings

¼ teaspoon salt
½ teaspoon chili powder
¼ teaspoon cayenne pepper
½ teaspoon turmeric
1½ pounds sweet potatoes (2 large or 3 medium), sliced into fry-size strips
1 tablespoon extra virgin olive oil
Lime wedges for serving

Preheat the oven to 450°F. Line a baking sheet with parchment paper.

In a small bowl, stir together the salt, chili powder, cayenne pepper, and turmeric.

In a large bowl, toss the sweet potatoes with the olive oil. Add the spice mixture and toss to coat.

Spread the sweet potatoes on the baking pan so the strips are not touching. (Use two pans if necessary.) Bake for 25 minutes. Flip the fries and bake for 15 to 20 minutes more, or until the fries are browned.

SMART AVOCADO BROWNIES WITH WALNUT BUTTER ICING

Can brownies be healthy? They can certainly be healthier. Here we have a little metabolic help from coconut oil, omega-3s from the eggs and walnut butter, potassium from the avocado, and fiber from the mung beans.

Makes 12 mini brownies

3 tablespoons organic virgin coconut oil, divided

1½ cups water

½ cup sprouted mung beans

½ avocado, peeled and pitted

¼ cup coconut sugar

3 organic omega-3 eggs

1 teaspoon baking powder

1 tablespoon vanilla extract

¼ cup unsweetened cocoa powder

Pinch Himalayan sea salt

¼ cup semisweet chocolate chips

Walnut butter for icing (optional)

Preheat the oven to 350°F.

Grease 12 mini-muffin cups with 1 tablespoon coconut oil.

Bring the water to a boil. Add the mung beans and boil for 4 minutes. Remove from the heat and drain. Let sit for 5 to 10 minutes.

Place the mung beans, avocado, coconut sugar, eggs, baking powder, vanilla, cocoa powder, sea salt, and 2 tablespoons coconut oil in a food processor and blend until smooth.

Add the chocolate chips and pulse until broken into tiny chocolate bits.

Pour the batter evenly into the greased mini-muffin cups and bake for 10 to 14 minutes.

Let cool, then "ice" lightly with walnut butter (if using).

LBT LINGO

Afternoon Ammunition: "Smart Snacks" that you can use to fight off urges for the candy bowl, vending machine, kids' snacks, and other food foes.

Anchor Behavior: The one food or exercise behavior you'll stick to without question when you travel. Put your Anchor Behavior in writing with the Glad Libs trip planner.

De-Bloaters: Foods that act in different manners to extinguish that extra layer of bloat. Asparagus and parsley are delicious de-bloaters.

Dunch: A larger lunch than dinner or an "entrée" lunch.

F-Its: Excuses for poor eating choices while traveling, such as "When I get home, I'll eat well," "Only a few more days," or any version of that. F-its when you're a little off give you license to eat more and worse. Cure the F-its with an Anchor Behavior reminder.

Food First-Aid Kit: Travel necessities that enable you to go on a trip of any duration and handle any situation with your weight loss plan unscathed. From jet lag to "plane puffies," there's a tonic for every travel trap. Don't leave home without it.

Food Pusher: Found in almost every family; mother-in-laws are commonly in this category. Food pushers have been known to ask, "Is that all you're eating?" or "How come you didn't try my potatoes?" Worst of all, they may plate food for you.

Menu Map: A meal plan for the week ahead that includes breakfast, lunch, and dinner options. There is a blank menu map (see page 36) and a sample completed week for you to reference (see page 42). Don't overcomplicate this; complicated can be a barrier.

No List: Foods that you should reject in order to be healthy and thin. Skim milk, bottled salad dressing, and cold cereal are all No list foods.

Nut Case: Nuts need to be portioned, and this handy gizmo beats digging into a giant container (a few times). Foodtrainers nut cases provide the right portion size and ground rules for nut quantities that you should stick to in order to make a smart start.

Obesogens: Chemicals potentially found in items such as personal care products and canned goods, as well as many forms of plastic, that may affect your weight. Use glass food containers and water bottles to steer clear of these sneaky substances.

One Plate Rule: The number one holiday planning tip and a good rule for any buffet situation. Before taking your food, observe the offerings and formulate your strategy. Savor this one plate of goodness because there are no second helpings in LBT.

OTID: The Other Twenty-three hours In the Day. Are you someone who does spin class each morning and then sits for the rest of the day? Sitting causes your body to redirect fat toward storage.

Overfruiting: Eating excess fruit; all excess sugar consumed can be warmly welcomed by your fat cells. Stick to one serving per day for weight loss.

Pre-Eating: A small amount of food consumed thirty to sixty minutes before a restaurant meal or party, especially if there will be alcohol. These pre-eaten calories will save you many more.

Pre-Snacktual Agreement: An agreement signed by midafternoon munchers contractually obligating you to pick two midafternoon snacks for the week ahead and stick to only those choices.

Reference Clothing: An item of clothing you remember feeling great in. Many people have "skinny jeans," but reference clothing can be a pair of fitted pants or a body-conscious dress. Men often use tuxedos for their reference clothing. Periodically try on your reference piece to gauge how you're doing.

Rule of 1 of 4: The number one restaurant eating rule is to choose only one of the following: bread, booze, dinner carb, or dessert—1 of 4, but no more.

Salad Accessories: Items that make salad eating fun, such as avocado, nuts, and olives. Contain your fun with only one accessory per salad for women, two for men.

Super Power Foods: Foods that go above and beyond regular foods. Super Power Foods are potent and effective. Hot sauce, teas, and coconut oil are Super Power Foods.

The 3 P's: Plan, Purchase, Prep (and Promise). Plan your weekly menu, pick an LBT recipe, map your menu, and make a shopping list. Only purchase items on the list. Prep a green, a grain, and a main. I promise you, this works.

Treat Training: Treats should be planned, portioned, and consumed socially; regular eating resumes with the next meal or snack.

Victory List: A list kept on your menu or in your phone with one LBT task you did well that day. Examples include "skipped the bread basket" or "had one liter of water by lunch."

The Walkthrough: A simple exercise done at the start of each day. Mentally walk yourself through the day ahead and plan your food, solving any diet dilemmas.

#TIDEI: stands for *tweet it, don't eat it*. Whether it's a holiday, a wedding day, or just another day, if you're on Twitter, I'm here for you. When you're tempted to get carried away, simply use the hashtag #TIDEI in a tweet to @Foodtrainers.

The following are food brands and kitchen tools that I recommend to make your journey to thin more delicious, satisfying, and easy. You may find many of these at your local market, or consult the websites provided.

BRAND	WEBSITE
Breakfast	
Cascadian Farm Frozen Berries	cascadianfarm.com
Cocomama Quinoa Cereal	cocomamafoods.com
Evolve Kefir	evolvekefir.com
Fage 2% Greek Yogurt	fageusa.com
Hemp Hearts	hemphearts.com
Living Fuel CocoChia Snack Mix	livingfuel.com
Siggi's Yogurt	skyr.com
SoCal Cleanse Protein	socalcleanse.com
Sunwarrior Protein	sunwarrior.com
Tera's Whey Protein	teraswhey.com
Condiments	
California Olive Ranch Oil	californiaoliveranch.com
Eden Apple Cider Vinegar	edenfoods.com

BRAND	WEBSITE
Jungle Products Virgin Coconut Oil	junglepi.com
Miso Master	great-eastern-sun.com
NuStevia	nunaturals.com
South River Miso Company	southrivermiso.com

Drinks

Amazing Grass Raw Reserve	amazinggrass.com
Eboost	eboost.com
Ayala's Herbal Water	herbalwater.com
Harmless Harvest Coconut Water	harmlessharvest.com
Harney and Son's Mother's Bouquet Tea	harney.com
Hint Water	drinkhint.com
Matcha Green Tea	domatcha.com
Pukka Night Time Valerian Tea	pukkaherbs.com
Synergy Kombucha	synergydrinks.com
Teas' Tea—Green Tea	teastea.com
Traditional Medicinals Fennel Tea	traditionalmedicinals.com
Yogi Detox Tea	yogiproducts.com

Fish

Cole's Sardines	colestrout.com/product/
Tonnino Jarred Tuna	tonnino.com
Vital Choice Salmon	vitalchoice.com/shop/pc/home.asp

Grains

Food for Life Ezekiel Sprouted Bread	foodforlife.com
French Meadow Sprouted Bread	frenchmeadow.com

BRAND	WEBSITE
Hilary's Veggie Burgers	hilaryseatwell.com
Orgran Crispibreads	orgran.com/home
Shiloh Farms Sprouted Bread	shilohfarms.com
Sunshine Burgers	sunshineburger.com
Vigilant Eats Oatmeal	vigilant-eats.com

Snacks

22 Days Bars	22daysnutrition.com
479° Popcorn	479popcorn.com/index.html
Almond Dream Bites	tastethedream.com
Annie Chun's Nori Snacks	anniechun.com/flavors/seaweed
Barney Butter	barneybutter.com
Beanitos	beanitos.com
Bubbies Pickles	bubbies.com
Food Should Taste Good Chips	foodshouldtastegood.com
GoGo Squeez	gogosqueez.com
Hail Merry Almonds	hailmerry.com
Health Warrior Bars	healthwarrior.com
Just Pure Foods Vegetable Chips	justpurefoods.com
Kind Bars	kindsnacks.com
Luna & Larry's Pops	coconutbliss.com
Mary's Gone Crackers	marysgonecrackers.com
NewTree Chocolate Spread	newtree.com/en_us
Oloves	oloves.com
Peeled Fruit Snacks	peeledsnacks.com
Sheffa Snack Mix	sheffafoods.com
SlantShack Jerky	slantshackjerky.com
SnackMasters Crackers	snackmasters.com
Sweet Riot Cacao Nibs	sweetriot.com

BRAND	WEBSITE
Way Better Snacks	gowaybetter.com
Yasso Pops	yasso.com
Zing Bars	zingbars.com

Pills

Carlson Vitamin D3 Drops	carlsonlabs.com
Nordic Naturals Ultimate Omega	nordicnaturals.com/consumers.php
Ultimate Flora	renewlife.com

Tools

Aero Speed Jump Rope	buddyleejumpropes.com
Black+Blum Lunch Pot	black-blum.com
Blender Bottle	blenderbottle.com
Eagle Creek Pack-It Cubes	shop.eaglecreek.com
EatSmart Floor Scales	eatsmartproducts.com
Fitbit	fitbit.com
FitKit	fitkit.com
Gaiam Balance Ball Chair	gaiam.com
Graze Organic Snack Bags	grazeorganic.com
Greenpan Cookware	westelm.com
Snapware Containers	snapware.com
Takeya	takeyausa.com
TRX Bands	trxtraining.com
Vitamix	vitamix.com
Withings Scales	withings.com

ACKNOWLEDGMENTS
OR MY TREATS

What would have happened if I had opened Foodtrainers in 2001 and nobody was interested? I am grateful for those first clients who sent a few more, and here we are thirteen years and thousands of clients later. Thank you for trusting me with your stories and for supporting me as I supported you. Without Foodtrainees, there would be no *Little Book of Thin*.

To Carolyn Brown: I am insanely lucky to have you on my team. I'm grateful for your nutrition nerd-dom, creativity, techie skills, and unparalleled thesaurusing. Thank you for not only helping with this project but caring about it (and me) too.

To Lauren Galit (and Caitlen at LKG Agency): Thank you for knowing I had a book in me. You listened to me spew ideas, and when I said, "It's all about planning," you looked up and said, "So that's the book." Thank you for championing this project, pushing me when things weren't quite there, and maintaining my voice throughout.

To the people at Perigee: I remember leaving that first meeting right after Hurricane Sandy. You described this "little book" you envisioned, providing readers with cheat sheets for every scenario. Thank you for making this a reality.

To my parents: Thank you for raising me in a home where a "snack" was a peach. You showed me that delicious meals and great books were two of the most important ingredients in life (eek, I hope you think this book is great).

To Louise, my kitchen partner and lifeline: Thank you for making sure there are family meals even when part of the family is at the office. I think you are an "adult-sitter" too.

And to all of you blog readers, I pinch myself when I look at Google Analytics and see that people are really reading my nutrition musings and heeding my suggestions. Via Twitter and Facebook, you've spread the Foodtrainers word and helped me see that I could reach beyond my office, so thank you.

INDEX

Page numbers in *italics* represent illustrations.

Abdominal fat, 57
Acai, 93
Acesulfame K, 18
Activity, 119–20
    foods, 56, 64, 104
After-dinner snacking, 60–61, 65
Afternoon snacking, 17,
    50–54, 142
Age-related weight gain, 112
Aggregate exercise, 113–14
Airplane food, 126–27
Airport food, 127, 128
Alcohol, 28, 145
    beer, 103–4
    blood sugar and, 85
    choosing best forms of, 92–93
    cocktails, 108, 145
    glassware for, 93
    lunch drinking, 129
    1 of 4 and no more rule, 87
    at Passover, 150
    substitute (rebound), 19
    during travel, 129
    at weddings and funerals, 156
    wine, 93
Allen, John, 55–56
*American Journal of Clinical
    Nutrition*, 57
Anchor behaviors, 126
Androgens, 15
Appetite hormone, 3
Apple cider vinegar, 140
Artificial sweeteners, 14, 18
Asparagus, 85
Aspartame, 18

Austerity days, 144
Avocado
    Drastic Salad with Avocado
        Dressing, 181–82
    Smart Avocado Brownies with
        Walnut Butter Icing, 190–91

Bacteria, 58
Bagels, 16, 151
Baking, 80–81
Batali, Mario, 33, 55
Batch cooking, 47–48
Beach, procedures to prepare for,
    133–42
Beef and Spinach "Green" Balls,
    185–86
Beer, 103–4
Beverages, 14, 24, 28, 93, 141
BHT, 18
Bikini Greenie, 179
Birthdays, 77–78, 109–10
Bisphenol A (BPA), 5
Bloating, 122, 135–36
Blood sugar, 85
Bobby Flay Fit, 86
Boiled eggs, 174
Boss, dining out at invitation
    of, 94–95
Bottled salad dressing, 17
BPA. *See* Bisphenol A
Braces, 64–65
Branson, Richard, 10
Bread, 21, 22
Breakfast, 2, 35, 142
Broccoli salad, 167

Broth, 44
Brown, Carolyn, 100
Brownies, 190–91
Brunch, 110–11
Buffet tactic, 156
Bullies, food, 106–7
Burgers
    Five Napkin Burger, 100
    Pesto Turkey Burgers, 182–83
Butter, 14, 145
    brownies with walnut, 190–91

Calories
    airplane meal, 127
    in beer, 103
    birthday parties and, 77
    in snacks, 54, 61, 104
    studies on, 62, 78
    timing of eating and, 62–63
    in tonic and coke, 92–93
Cancer, 91
Candy, 61, 63
Carbohydrates, 21–22, 25, 87
    portion size for, 29–30
    soybean, 91
    in specific cuisines, 88, 89
Cardio, 9–10
Cathy cartoon, 161
Cereal, 16, 104
Chamomile, 8
Cheat day, 69
Cheat sheet, 24–28, 141
Checklist, 10–11
Cheese, 29
Chicken, 105
    broth, 44
    "Greek" Curried Chicken
        Salad, 173
    Souper Easy Chicken Soup, 172
    Starter Chicken Cutlets, 171
Children
    baking with, 80–81
    birthday parties, 77–78
    game day, 81
    menus for, 82–83
    packing lunch for, 79
Child's pose, 139
Chocolate, 18
Christmas, 152
Cilantro, 138
CLA. See Conjugated linoleic acid
Closed Kitchen, 8, 61, 63–65, 140

Cocktails, 108, 145
Coconut oil, 45, 140
Coke, 92–93
Cold cereal, 16
Colors, 18
Comments, from friends, 159–60
Condiments, 27
Conjugated linoleic acid (CLA), 14
Constipation, vacation, 123
Container eating, 55, 96
Cookies, 66–67
Cooking, 33
    in batches, 47–48
    vegetable cooking times, 176
Cornell study, on men's view
    of overweight women, 99
Crackers, quinoa, 35
Cravings, 58–59
Criticism, 147–48
Crunchy foods, 56
Curfew, electronic, 9. See also
    Closed Kitchen
Cutlets, chicken, 171
Cydylo, Katrina, 139

Dairy, 15
Dancing, 156
Date-Night Salmon, 187–88
Dating, 98–102
Day drinking, 129
De-bloating foods, 135–36
Denver airport, 128
Dessert, 60–61, 87. See also Sweets
Detox powder, 140
Diced tomatoes, 44
Diet food, 14
Dieting, myths about, 67
Dinner
    after-dinner snacking,
        60–61, 65
    after-dinner teas, 8
    as endpoint, 63
    family and dinnertime,
        78–79
    parties, 68–69
    planning, 39–40
    pre-beach sample, 142
Doctor's orders, 94–95
Dominican University, 51–52
Double-header, exercise, 117
Drastic procedures, pre-beach,
    133–42

Drastic Salad with Avocado
    Dressing, 181–82
Dressing, salad, 17, 181–82
Drinking. *See* Alcohol
Duhigg, Charles, 73
Dunch, 7–8, 38

Eagle Creek, 125
Easter, 150–51
Eating. *See also* Foods; Snacking;
    Timing
    emotional, 117–18
    fast, 86
    at friend's house, 68–69
    new relationships and eating
        habits, 100–102
    out of containers, 55, 96
    pre-, 85
    procrastinating
        (procrastinEATING),
        154, 156
Eggs
    boiled, 174
    Green Eggs, 35, 169
Emotional eating, 117–18
Essential Poached Salmon, 186–87
Exercise, 19
    age-related weight gain and, 112
    aggregate, 113–14
    double header, 117
    fitness apps for, 130
    Foodtrainers exercise dream
        week, *116*
    goals, 114, 130
    during holidays, 153
    planning, 114–15
    snacks before and after, 118–19
    during travel, 129–30
    variety, 115, 117
    weekly cardio, 9–10
    workout tips and myths, 119–20
    in workplace, 120

Family, 76–83. *See also* Children
    dinnertime, 78–79
    game day snacks, 81
    parenthood challenges, 76
Fast eating, 86
Fat
    abdominal, 57
    study on timing, calories
        and, 62

Fats, 23–24
    fat-free foods, 14, 15
    list of healthy, 26–27
    in milk, 15
FDA, 5
Fermented foods, 58–59, 90–91
First-aid kit, food and travel,
    122–25, *124*
Fish. *See also* Salmon
    eco-friendly, 5–6
    No-Fuss Fish, 188–89
    as restaurant choice, 85–86
Fitbits, 120
FitChickNYC, 115
FitKit, 130
Fitness apps, 130
F-its, 131
Five Napkin Burger, 100
Flavorings, 27
Flay, Bobby, 86
Flex Areas, 126
Food bullies, 106–7
Food court, 128
Food-free hours, 8, 62–63
Foodnetwork.com, 86
Food pushers, 147
Foods. *See also* Holidays; *specific
    cuisines*
    activity, 56, 64, 104
    airline, 126–27
    airport, 127, 128
    crunchy, 56
    de-bloating, 135–36
    diet, 14
    to eliminate before beach, 135
    fermented, 58–59, 90–91
    live, 22
    picks of children's, 82
    politely refusing, 147
    promise, 33
    to satisfy cravings for sweets,
        58–59
    shared fare situations, 107–9
    staple, 44–46
    super power, 140, 141
    travel first-aid kit, 122–25, *124*
    what-to-eat cheat sheet,
        24–28, 141
Foodtrainers, 1, 6, 23, 50, 134
    exercise dream week, *116*
    favorite alcoholic beverage, 93
    lament, 49

Foodtrainers (*cont.*)
  menu map, 36–37, 42–43
  on Twitter, 63, 157
Fourth of July, 151
French green lentils, 184
Friends, comments from, 159–60
Fries, sweet potato, 189–90
Frittatas, 35, 169
Frozen yogurt, 16–17
Fruit, 6, 23, 26, 141. *See also*
    Smoothies
  portion size for, 30
Funerals, 155–56

Game day, 81
Garlic, 44–45
Genetically modified organisms
    (GMOs), 91
Ghrelin, 2, 44
Glad Libs, *132*
Glassman, Keri, 128
Glassware, 93
Gluten, 22
GMOs. *See* Genetically modified
    organisms
Gone with the Wind, 98
Grains, 6–7, 45, 46, 141
  sprouted, 22
Greek yogurt, 35, 173
Green Eggs, 35, 169
Greens, 46, 85–86
Green tea, 5, 178
Guilt, 67, 70–71, 72
Gum, 17–18
Gumbel, Bryant, 102
Gussow, Joan, 15

Hall of shame, 150–52
Halloween, 151
Hamburgers, 105. *See also* Burgers
Hanukkah, 152
Happy hour, 129
Harney and Son's Mother's
    Boutique tea, 64
Harvard School of Public Health,
    6–7
Healthy eating habits, 100–102
Hemp, 140, 180
Higgs, Suzanne, 63–64
Hoff, Amie, 114
Holidays
  exercise during, 153

hall of shame, 150–52
honesty and criticism during,
    147–48
one-plate rule, 148, 152–53
problem solving for specific,
    143–45, 147–48, 152–56
treats, 146–47
Hormones
  appetite, 3
  disrupters, 5
  hunger, 2, 44
  skim milk creating male, 15
  soy influence on, 91
Hors d'oeuvres, 144–45
Hot dogs, 105
Hot sauce, 44
Hunger hormone, 2, 44
Hydration helpers, 4
Hydrogenated starch
    hydrolysates, 18

Indian food, 88
Invisalign, 64–65
Isoflavones, 90

Jet lag, 122
Juice
  Bikini Greenie, 179
  Juicy snacks, 138–39

Kale
  Kale Slaw, 170
  Starter Kale, 168
Karan, Donna, 51
Kids. *See* Children
Kitchen, closed, 8, 61,
    63–65, 140
Kombucha, 59

Latkes, 152
Lentils, 45
  Super Bowl Stew, 184
Leptin, 3
Liquid snacks, 28
Live food, 22
Live with Regis and Kelly, 102
Ludwig, David, 6
Lunch, 38–39. *See also* Dunch
  brunch and, 110–11
  children's packed, 79
  lunch-time drinking, 129
  pre-beach sample, 142

Madison Square Garden, 106
Main dishes, preparing ahead
    for, 47
Maintenance, 163–64
Makes-You-Pee Tea, 136, 140
Mannitol, 18
Martinis, 93
Massive Health, 51
Matcha Colada, 178
Matzo, 144
Meatballs, beef and spinach,
    185–86
Mednick, Sara, 57–58
Menu. *See also* Planning
    for children's meals, 82–83
    children's restaurant, 82–83
    map, 36–37, 42–43
    online, 84–85
    planning, 35–40
    pre-beach sample, 142
Mercury, 138
Mexican food, 88–89
Milk, 15
Miso, 58–59
    Miso Broccoli and Quinoa
        Salad, 167

Napping, 57, 60
New York Times, 71
Nighttime teas, 64
No-Fuss Fish, 188–89
No's, 12, 13–19. *See also*
    Rebounds, for no's
NuStevia, 14
Nutrition bars, 57
Nuts, 26–27, 31

OA. *See* Overeaters Anonymous
Obesogens, 5, 21
Office presentation scenario,
    66–67
Oils, 23, 45, 140
Olive oil, 45
Omega-3s, 3, 5, 23–24, 174
1 of 4 and no more rule, 86–88
One-plate rule, 148, 152–53, 156
Onions, 44–45
Orthodontia, 64–65
Other Twenty-three hours In the
    Day (OTID), 119–20, 130
Overeaters Anonymous (OA), 61
Overeating, 49

Packed lunch, 79
Packing cubes, 125. *See also* Travel
Pantry staples, 44–46
Papain, 178
Parenthood, 76
Passover, 150
Pedometers, 120
Peeps, 150
Peer pressure, 106–7
Pesto Turkey Burgers, 182–83
Picks of kids' food, 82
Pizza, 94
Planning, 32–40, 42–46
    afternoon snack, 51–52
    breakfast, 35
    dinner, 39–40
    for disparagement, 148
    exercise, 114–15
    food-related questions for, 74
    lunch, 38–39
    menu map, 36–37, 42–43
    pantry staples, 44–46
    restaurant game plan, 84–96
    treat, 68–69
    walkthrough, 72–75
    witching hour and, 49
Plastic water bottles, 5
Pops, 17
Portions, 28–31
    carbohydrate, 29–30
    holidays and, 147
    for nuts, 31
    overview of, 31
    protein, 29
    takeout ordering and,
        95–96
    treat, 69–70
Positivity, 158–59
Post, Emily, 94
Potassium, 136
Potatoes, sweet potato fries,
    189–90
Praise, 158–59
Pre-beach procedures, 133–42
Pre-eating, 85
Preparation, 46–47
Pre-Snacktual Agreement,
    51–52, 53
Probiotics, 58, 59
Problem solving, holiday, 143–45,
    147–48, 152–56
ProcrastinEATING, 154, 156

Promise, 47, 51–52
    foods, 33
Protein, 20–21
    breakfast, 2
    exercise and, 118
    in Greek yogurt, 35
    list of choices, 24–25
    portion size, 29
    powder, 140, 177, 178
    pre-beach, 140, 141
    smart snacking and, 54
    in smoothies, 177
    snack, 119
    soy protein isolates and TVP, 90
    in sprouted grains, 22
Pu-erh tea, 59
Pukka, 64
Pumpkin seeds, 57
Purchasing, 40–46

Questions, food-related, 74
Quinoa, 16, 46
    crackers, 35
    Miso Broccoli and Quinoa
        Salad, 167
    Spinach-Quinoa Cakes, 166
    Starter Quinoa, 165–66

Rebounds, for no's
    alcohol, 19
    bagels, 16
    cold cereal, 16
    dairy, 15
    fat-free foods, 14
    frozen yogurt, 17
    gum, 17–18
    salad dressing, 17
    soda, 14
Relationships, new, 100–102
Replacements. See Rebounds,
    for no's
Restaurants, 84–96
    alcohol choices at, 92–93
    boss invitations to, 94–95
    children's menus at, 82–83
    online menu and, 84–85
    pre-eating before going to, 85
    problem areas, 86–87
    rule 1 of 4 and no more, 86–88
    takeout ordering, 95–96
Resting metabolic rate (RMR), 112
Rice, 46

RMR. See Resting metabolic rate
Road rules, 128–32
Rosh Hashanah, 151
Roth, Geneen, 70

Salad
    accessories, 27, 89, 92
    Drastic Salad with Avocado
        Dressing, 181–82
    dressing, 17, 181, 182
    "Greek" Curried Chicken
        Salad, 173
    Kale Slaw, 170
    Miso Broccoli and Quinoa
        Salad, 167
    ordering with pizza, 94
    restaurant, 89, 92
    sex and, 102
Salk Institute, 62
Salmon
    for breakfast, 35
    Date-Night Salmon, 187–88
    Essential Poached Salmon,
        186–87
Salt, 45
SamePlate.com, 101
Scales, 161–63
School of Public Health,
        Harvard, 6–7
Sea salt, 45
Second brain, 58
Seeds, 23–24, 26–27, 57
Self-compassion, 72
Seltzer, 92–93
Sex, salad and, 102
Shakes, 180
Shape.com survey, 61–62
Shared fare, 107–9
Shopping, 40–42
SIRT1, 8
6 p.m. SoCal Shake, 180
Ski jacket snack, 123
Skim milk, 15
Skinny gene (SIRT1), 8
Slaw, kale, 170
Sleep, 9, 65
Smart Avocado Brownies with
        Walnut Butter Icing, 190–91
Smoothies. See also Shakes
    breakfast, 35
    Matcha Colada, 178
    Starter Smoothie, 177

Snacking
    after-dinner, 60–61, 65
    afternoon, 17, 50–54, 142
    Pre-Snacktual Agreement,
        51–52, 53
Snacks
    calories in, 61, 104
    before and after exercise,
        118–19
    game day, 81
    juicy, 138–39
    liquid, 28
    protein, 119
    restaurant pre-eating, 85
    ski jacket, 123
    smart, 54–57
    sports and, 81, 104–5
    stadium, 104
    after treat, 71–72
Snoozing, 57, 60
SoCal Cleanse, 140, 180
Socializing, 97–111
    balanced, 97–98
    birthday, 109–10
    brunch, 110–11
    dating, 98–99
    peer pressure and food bullies,
        106–7
    shared fare situations,
        107–9
    sports and, 103–6
Soda, 14
Sorbitol, 18
Soups, chicken, 172
Soy, 18, 90–91
Special K, 33, 48
Spices, 45
Spicy Sweet Potato Fries, 189–90
Spinach
    Beef and Spinach "Green" Balls,
        185–86
    Spinach-Quinoa Cakes, 166
Sports, 81, 103–6
Sprouted grains, 22
Stadium snacks, 104
Staples, 44–46
Starbucks, 73
Starchy vegetables, 23
Starter Chicken Cutlets, 171
Starter Kale, 168
Starter Quinoa, 165–66
Starter Smoothie, 177

Steak
    ways to turn down, 94–95
    Weekday Tenderloin, 183
Steamed vegetables, 175–76
Stew, 184
Strategic shopping guidelines, 40–41
Strip-strategy game, 148
Substitutes. See Rebounds, for no's
Sugar substitutes, 63
Sunflower seeds, 57
Super Bowl, 103, 104, 106
Super Bowl Stew, 184
Super Power Foods, 140, 141
Supplements, probiotic, 59
Support, 61
Sushi, 89
Sweeteners, artificial, 14, 18
Sweet potatoes, fries made with,
    189–90
Sweets. See also Dessert; Treats
    foods to satisfy cravings for,
        58–59
    as reward, 66–67
Swift, Taylor, 19
Swimsuits, 133, 137, 179

Table salt, 45
Takeout, 95–96
Teas
    after dinner, 8
    fermented, 59
    green, 5, 178
    Makes-You-Pee Tea, 136, 140
    nighttime, 64
    travel, 127
Television, 63–64
Tenderloin, 183
Ten Steps to Svelte, 1–11
    checklist, 11
Textured vegetable protein
    (TVP), 90
Thanksgiving, 145, 146, 151–52
Thin-I-Gette Dressing, 181
3 P's, 34–48
    planning, 32–40, 42–46
    preparation, 46–47
    purchasing, 40–46
Time zones, 127
Timing, 62–63
    breakfast, 2
    food-free hours and, 8, 62–63
    witching hour, 49, 51, 60–61

Tofu, 91
Tomatoes, 44
Tonic water, 92–93
Travel
    alcohol drinking during, 129
    days or daze, 126–27
    delaying treats strategy, 130–31
    exercise during, 129–30
    F-its, 131
    Food First-Aid Kit, 122–25, *124*
    Glad Libs, *132*
    packing checklist, 130
    packing cubes, 125
    pre- and post-trip menu, 125
    road rules for, 128–32
    tea and water for, 127
Treats, 66–68
    choosing best version of, 82
    do-it-yourself, 75
    guilt-free, 70–71
    holiday, 146–47
    meal or snack after, 71–72
    planned, 68–69
    portioned, 69–70
    socially consumed, 70–71
    training, 68–72
    travel strategy of delaying,
        130–31
Truths, 37, 43
Tummy turbulence, 123
Turkey burgers, 182–83
TVP. *See* Textured vegetable
    protein
Twist, 139
Twitter, 63, 157

Umbrella drinks, 92
Unbuttoning, 148, 153
Uniform snacker, 51
University of Birmingham, 63

Vacation, constipation
        during, 123

Valentine's Day, 150
Vegetables, 96
    aversion to, 101
    broth, 44
    list of choices, 25–26
    misconception about, 175
    portion size for, 30
    starchy, 23
    Starter Smoothie, 177
    steamed, 175–76
Victory list, 158–59
Vinegar, 45–46, 140
Virgin Group, 10
Vitamin D, 3
Vodka, 93

Walking, 153
Walkthrough, 72–75
Wall Street Journal, 129
Walnuts, in brownies, 190–91
Wansink, Brian, 70
Water, 4, 127, 139–40
    bottles, 5
Weddings, 155–56
Weekday Tenderloin, 183
Weighing, 161–63
Weight gain
    age-related, 112
    Cornell study on, 99
    television linked with,
        63–64
Whey powder, 177, 178
White bread, 22
Whole Foods Days, 125, *132*
Willett, Walter, 15
Wine, 93
Wings, 105
Witching hour, 49, 51, 60–61
Workouts. *See* Exercise

Yoga, 117–18, 139
Yogurt, 14, 16–17, 35, 173
Yom Kippur, 151

ABOUT THE AUTHOR

Lauren Slayton received her undergraduate degree in sociology from Tulane University with honors and a master's degree in clinical nutrition from New York University. She worked at St. Luke's-Roosevelt obesity research unit and was a nutritionist at Equinox fitness clubs prior to opening Foodtrainers, a nutritional consultancy specializing in weight management and sports nutrition, in 2001.

Aside from one-on-one counseling, Slayton lectures on topics ranging from running and weight to organics 101 for running groups, schools, and corporations. She has written for and been quoted in articles for numerous websites, magazines, and television programs, including *Allure*, *Marie Claire*, *Cosmopolitan*, *InStyle*, *Cooking Light*, *Harper's Bazaar*, *Hamptons*, *Self*, *Fitness*, WebMD, the *New York Post*, *The Daily Show with Jon Stewart*, ABC's *Eyewitness News*, *The Early Show*, Fox News, and *Good Morning America*.

An avid runner, tennis player, and skier, she lives, eats, and exercises in New York City with her husband, Marc; her sons, Myles and Weston; and her much-beloved and well-used Vitamix.

Contact the author online:

Foodtrainers.com
Blog: Foodtrainers.blogspot.com
Pinterest: Foodtrainers.blogspot.com/Pinterest
Twitter: @Foodtrainers
Facebook: Foodtrainers